Bedtime Stories for Psychiatry Residents

Psychiatry Board Review Topics A to Z

Bascom K. Bradshaw, DO, MPH, MAS

Dedication

To my wife, Tracy, and our son, Felix, the Sweetest-P.

To my parents, Delbert and Mary Bradshaw.

I would also like to thank (in no particular order) Izzy, Scarlet, Baby Tupac, Frisco, Dingo, Mustafa, Peter, Tom-Tom, Yoda, Tux, Flynn, George, Bruno, Cappuccino, Millie, Jak-Jak, Big Louie, and in memory of Ozzy and Princess.

Abbreviations

ADHD	Attention-Deficit Hyperactivity Disorder
AED	antiepileptic drug
ASPD	Antisocial Personality Disorder
a/w	associated with
b/t	between
CNS	central nervous system
d/o	disorder(s)
d/t	due to
dx	diagnosis
dz	disease
EEG	electroencephalogram
EPS	extrapyramidal symptoms
FDA	U.S. Food and Drug Administration
GBS	Guillain-Barre Syndrome
GERD	gastroesophageal reflux
hx	history
IQ	intelligence quotient
MDD	Major Depressive Disorder
MI	myocardial infarction
NMS	neuroleptic malignant syndrome
PD	personality disorder
PET	positron emission tomography
PTSD	posttraumatic stress disorder

SPECT	single photon emission computed tomography
sxs	symptoms
TD	tardive dyskinesia
tx	treatment
w/	with
w/o	with out

Introduction

Welcome to *Bedtime Stories for Psychiatry Residents*. This study guide is not an exhaustive review for the American Osteopathic Board of Neurology and Psychiatry and American Board of Psychiatry and Neurology psychiatry board examinations. The goal of this study guide is to supplement a guided reading program using up-to-date references.

This guide is intended to be a casual review of psychiatry board topics that I have encountered while reviewing for the psychiatry boards, as well as discussions stemming from clinical encounters during my residency training; it should be used in conjunction with other study aids. The topics can be reviewed in any order but have been arranged in alphabetical order for ease of locating topics.

It is suggested that the reader review a couple topics each day. Your review should include writing down everything you know about the topic; compare your notes with the bolded items under each topic heading. The reader can also use this guide to quickly skim through topics. The random nature of topic headings in this book is to stimulate further reading in reference books and electronic resources. By doing this, the reader should explore related material for a better understanding of the topic in a larger context.

People say, you must have been the class clown. And I say, No, I wasn't.
But I sat next to the class clown, and I studied him.

-Dr. Pearl, *Waiting for Guffman*, 1996

A

Absence seizure initial treatment

-Opinions vary about how to rank medications

-U.S. expert opinion, order of preference is **ethosuximide**, *then* valproic acid, and lamotrigine (Wheless et al. 2005)

-European expert opinion prefers to rank valproic acid first, followed by ethosuximide, and finally lamotrigine (Wheless et al. 2007)

-Cochrane Review reports that there is insufficient evidence to inform clinical practice (Posner et al. 2005)

-International League against Epilepsy (ILAE), noted a marked paucity of published data from adequately powered, seizure-type–specific studies (Glauser et al. 2006)

Absence vs. Partial complex seizures

-**abrupt ending** of typical absence seizures, **w/o postictal phase**, is *most* useful clinical feature in distinguishing the 2 conditions

Partial Complex

-aura is often

-consciousness is *impaired*

-movements are usually simple, repetitive but may include complex activity

-postictal behavior; amnesia, confusion, and tendency to sleep

-frequency; 1-2 per week

-duration; 2-3 minutes

-precipitants; none identified

-EEG w/ spikes and polyspike and waves, usually over both temporal regions

-AED tx; carbamazepine, phenytoin

Absence Seizure

-aura does NOT typically occur

-consciousness is *lost at onset*

-movements include blinking and facial and finger automatisms (duration dependent)

-**NO postictal abnormality** except amnesia for ictus

-frequency; several daily

-duration; 1-10 seconds

-precipitants; hyperventilation, photic stimulation

-EEG w/ generalize 3 Hz spike-and-wave complexes

-AED tx; ethosuxamide, valproate

Acculturation; risk for suicide, substance abuse, alcoholism
-individuals who assume a **new cultural identity** *consonant w/* that of the **host culture**

-individuals *may be* at **higher risk for suicide, substance abuse**, and **alcoholism** if he or she **abandons native culture** but *does NOT incorporate* **behaviors and values of the host culture**

Acute dystonia and haloperidol
-occurs *most commonly* during the **week after initiation of antipsychotics** or following an **abrupt and rapid dose increase** (Ayd 1961; Barnes and Spence 2000; Remington and Kapur 1996)

-occurs most commonly in **children and young adults**, especially in **males**

-may appear as torticollis, trismus, tongue protrusion, pharyngeal constriction, laryngospasm, blepharospasm, oculogyric crisis, or abnormal contractions of any part of the body

-may complain of tongue thickening, throat tightening, and difficulty speaking or swallowing

-acute tx w/either anticholinergic agent or antihistamine is usually highly effective

-may need to be repeated at intervals if acute dystonia recurs before the dose of the anticholinergic is stabilized

-medications may need to be given parenterally if respiratory difficulty develops

Adoption studies, role of environment in behavioral genetics

-based on knowledge that adoption **separates 2 major influences**, **genes** and **rearing**

-provides naturalistic setting w/ ideal separation of genetic factors from environmental influences

-4 types of adoption studies:

Adoptee study method

-study of adopted-away children of parent w/ disorder

Cross-fostering strategy

-study of children born of non-disordered parents adopted into family w/ disordered parent

Adoptees' family method

-study of adoptive and biological relatives of disordered adoptees

Monozygotic twins reared apart

-study of monozygotic twins reared apart

-adoption studies have been carried out for schizophrenia, mood d/o, alcoholism, drug abuse, sociopathy, ADHD, other psychiatric conditions; IQ and personality variables

Aggressive behavior in preschool children; verbal inability

-children behave aggressively for many reasons

-may NOT have anything to do w/ child rearing

-young children do NOT have good language skills compared to older children

-children *may act* **aggressively** if he or she feels helpless and is **unable to express feelings verbally**

-children generally understand language better than they can use it; children should be spoken to in **age-appropriate language** about why it is important not to hit others

-**role-playing may be helpful**; child should be encouraged to use the language that he does have at his disposal to express his feelings to others

Akathisia, clinical features

-**subjective feeling** of **motor restlessness**, compelling need to be in constant movement; may be seen as extrapyramidal adverse effect from antipsychotic use

-may be mistaken for psychotic agitation

-tx includes **discontinuing medication** causing akathisia; **beta-adrenergic receptor antagonists** (propanolol considered drug of choice), **benzodiazepines**, and **clonidine**

-trial of **anticholinergics** (cyproheptadine, benztropine) for tx neuroleptic-induced acute akathisia is reasonable

Alcohol intoxication and suicide risk assessment

-patients under the influence of alcohol or other substances are at an **increased risk of causing harm to themselves or others**, often accidentally or impulsively

-*should* generally *NOT be* **discharged** from psychiatric emergency service into less restrictive setting unless he or she has attained clinical **sobriety**

-clinical sobriety is NOT to be equated w/ a particular blood concentration of intoxicant

-patient should be retained for additional observation; should focus on erratic behaviors

-duration of observation will be a *function* of pharmacokinetics of circulating drug

Alcohol intoxication, clinical presentation

-degree of **clinical impairment** from alcohol intoxication is dependent on the individual's **tolerance**; **amount** and **type** of alcoholic beverage ingested; **amount absorbed**

-blood alcohol level of **0.4 g/dL** is a/w **50% mortality risk** in **nonalcoholic** persons

-rule of thumb is that the body metabolizes ~ **1 drink** (~ 0.015 g/dL) **per hour**

Clinical sxs of alcohol intoxication in **nontolerant** patient

Blood alcohol level (mg/dL)	Clinical symptoms
30	Attention difficulties (mild), euphoria
50	Coordination problems, driving is legally impaired
100	Ataxia, drunk driving
200	Confusion, decreased consciousness
> 400	**Anesthesia**, possible **coma**, possible **death**

Alcohol Withdrawal, delirium tremens

-withdrawal typically *begins* **6-8 hours after last drink**, *peaks* **24-28 hours after last drink**; generally resolves w/in 7 days (Myrick and Anton 2004)

-only ~5% of individuals w/ alcohol dependence will develop more than mild to moderate withdrawal sxs

-alcohol hallucinosis occurs in 3-10% of patients w/ severe alcohol withdrawal

-can present as auditory, visual, or tactile hallucinations in presence of clear sensorium

-delirium tremens (DT), or alcohol withdrawal delirium, is characterized by agitation and tremulousness, autonomic instability, fevers, auditory and visual hallucinations, and disorientation

-DT usually develops 2-4 days from last drink; average duration < 1 week

-DT has been estimated to occur in 5% of patients admitted for alcohol withdrawal (Mayo-Smith et al. 2004)

-considered a medical emergency; **mortality rate** can be as high as **20% w/o prompt and adequate tx of severe withdrawal**

-**seizures** are estimated to occur in **5-15% of patients**; usually **occur in first 24 hours from last drink**, but can occur **any time in first 5 days**

-alcohol withdrawal seizures are usually grand mal in type

-**past hx of alcohol withdrawal seizures** are at **increased risk for seizures** in subsequent episodes of alcohol withdrawal

Alcohol-induced "blackout"

-**anterograde amnesia** for events of any part of drinking episode w/o loss of consciousness; unable to make new long term memories, but still able to retrieve the memories established before alcohol consumption

-characterized by memory impairment during intoxication in relative absence of other skill deficits

-NOT to be confused w/ "passing out"

-may be **complete (en-bloc)** or **partial (fragmentary, or grayout)**

-en bloc blackout is complete amnesia for significant events otherwise memorable under usual circumstances; defining characteristic is permanent memory loss for period and cannot be recalled under any circumstances

-fragmentary blackouts occur more frequently; recall is usually possible and can be aided by cueing

-no longer considered as a signal of irreversible alcoholism

Alcohol-Induced Amnestic Disorder, Korsakoff's syndrome

-essential feature of alcohol-induced persisting amnestic d/o is disturbance in short-term memory caused by prolonged heavy use of alcohol

-rare in persons younger than age 35

-also described as Wernicke-Korsakoff Syndrome (a set of acute sxs) and Korsakoff's syndrome (chronic condition)

Wernicke's encephalopathy

-**completely reversible w/ tx**; only ~ 20% of patients w/Korsakoff's syndrome recover

-pathophysiological connection b/w 2 syndromes is **thiamine deficiency**, caused either by **poor nutritional habits** or by **malabsorption** problems

-thiamine is a cofactor for several important enzymes; may be involved in conduction of axon potential along axon and in synaptic transmission

-neuropathological lesions are **symmetrical** and **paraventricular**, involving mammillary bodies, thalamus, hypothalamus, midbrain, pons, medulla, fornix, and cerebellum

-tx in early stages of Wernicke's encephalopathy responds rapidly to large doses of parenteral thiamine; believed to be effective in preventing progression into Korsakoff's syndrome; dosage of thiamine is usually initiated at 100 mg by mouth 2-3 times daily and is continued for 1 to 2 weeks

-in patients w/ alcohol-related disorders who are receiving IV glucose solution, it is good practice to include 100 mg of thiamine in each liter of the glucose solution

Korsakoff's syndrome

-**chronic amnestic** syndrome that *can follow* Wernicke's encephalopathy

-cardinal features are **impaired mental syndrome** (especially **recent memory**) and **anterograde amnesia** in an **alert and responsive** patient; may or may not have confabulation

-tx of Korsakoff's syndrome is also thiamine given 100 mg by mouth 2-3 times daily; should continue for 3-12 months; few patients ever fully recover, although many have some **improvement in cognitive abilities** w/ **thiamine** and **nutritional support**

-Korsakoff's syndrome can occur in other malnourished conditions, such as marasmus, gastric carcinoma, and HIV

Alexia w/ agraphia; embolic stroke, left angular gyrus
-alexia w/ agraphia is also known as **angular gyrus syndrome** and **central alexia**

-considered **acquired illiteracy**; patients **lose previously acquired reading and writing skills**

-*most* **lose spelling** and *ability to understand words* **spelled to them**

-many patients have **fluent, paraphasic speech**, unlike preserved speech of pure alexia w/o agraphia

-**auditory comprehension** is *much superior* to reading comprehension

-lesion usually involves **angular gyrus area in LEFT inferior parietal lobule**

-syndrome was described by Dejerine

-closely related to pure alexia w/ agraphia syndrome, Gerstmann syndrome; Gerstmann brought together 4 deficits of agraphia, acalculia, right-left confusion, and finger agnosia and associated them w/ lesions of dominant parietal lobe; alexia was not originally a cardinal feature of Gerstmann syndrome but is often associated

-modern authors (Benton) have questioned validity of Gerstmann syndrome

-some patients may have one or more deficits w/o the others; stimulation studies in epileptic patients have reproduced combinations of these deficits w/ stimulation in angular gyrus area, confirming association of key elements of Gerstmann syndrome

Alzheimer Disease, early onset

-some forms of **familial early-onset** Alzheimer dz can appear *as early as* **third decade**; represents a subgroup of **< 10% of all familial cases** of Alzheimer dz

-**familial forms of Alzheimer dz** account for **< 7% of all cases of Alzheimer dz**; most cases are sporadic (not inherited)

-**mutations** in genes coding for **3 proteins** unequivocally cause Alzheimer dz:

amyloid precursor protein (APP, on chromosome **21**)

presenilin I (on chromosome **14**)

presenilin II (on chromosome **1**)

-all lead to a relative **excess in production** of **stickier 42-amino acid** form of **beta-amyloid** peptide over less sticky 40-amino acid form

Alzheimer's Disease, dementia

-**most common** cause of dementia in patients *over* **age 65**

-**definite** dx requires **histologic** examination of brain tissue

-probable, or clinical, dx includes: **insidious onset** of a progressively **worsening dementia**; clinical and laboratory evaluations that exclude alternative neurologic and systemic illness

-above clinical criteria yields an antemortem diagnostic accuracy of **almost 90%**; would be more reliable by excluding those w/ EPS and frontal lobe dysfunction

Amantadine, treatment of antipsychotic side effects, Parkinsonism

-FDA-approved for **tx of neuroleptic-induced Parkinsonism** (NIP) and Parkinson's dz, as well as tx and prophylaxis of influenza A respiratory illness; NOT effective in tx of akathisia

-dosages of **100-300 mg/day** are used for tx of NIP, and plasma concentrations may have some correlation w/ improvement

-water-soluble tricyclic amine; binds to M2 protein, membrane protein that functions as an ion channel on influenza A virus

-activity in reducing EPS is not known; shown to be **active at glutamate receptors**

-slowly and well absorbed from GI tract, w/ unchanged oral bioavailability over dose range of 50-300mg

-reaches steady state in 4-7 days; plasma concentrations (0.12-1.12 g/mL) may have some correlation w/ improvement in EPS

-relatively constant blood levels and long duration of action; excreted unchanged by kidneys

-half-life for elimination is ~16 hrs; prolonged in elderly patients and in impaired renal function

-has no anticholinergic activity in animal tests, only 1/209,000th as potent as atropine

-appears to cause release of dopamine and other catecholamines from intraneuronal storage sites in amphetamine-like mechanism; also shown to have activity at glutamate receptors, which may contribute to its antiparkinsonian effect

-no reported interactions b/w amantadine and other drugs

Anosognosia

-**failure to recognize** a **deficit** or **dz**

-**most common** example is **ignoring a left hemiparesis** because of a **right cerebral infarction**

-another example is **denial of blindness** from occipital lobe infarction (**Anton's syndrome**)

Antipsychotic use in elderly

-*increasingly* used in geriatric patients, particularly dementia given difference in prevalence rates; prevalence of schizophrenia remains < 1%, prevalence of dementia is ~2-5% for people > 60 yrs, increases to 15-40% for > 85 yrs

-**not FDA-approved** for tx of psychosis or behavioral dyscontrol in **dementia**

-drug interactions need to be considered in elderly patients

-age-related **decreases in gut motility** and **anticholinergic effects** of antipsychotics may decrease absorption rates

-antipsychotic drugs undergo **biotransformation primarily in the liver**, w/ GI tract, lungs, and kidneys being secondary sites; antipsychotics have slightly **longer half-lives in elderly**; drugs take **longer to reach therapeutic blood levels** and **longer to leave the system**

-dopamine neurons degenerate w/ aging, particularly after 70 yrs, **decrease in number** of available **dopaminergic receptors** *reduces tolerance* of elderly patients to antipsychotics, thereby increasing likelihood of neurological side effects, including EPS and TD

-more sensitive to side effects, **sedation**, **cardiac** effects (e.g., tachycardia, orthostatic hypotension), **anticholinergic** side effects (e.g., dry mouth, blurred vision, constipation, urinary retention), **NMS** w/ hyperpyrexia, **autonomic instability** and tachycardia, pigmentary retinopathy, weight gain and associated metabolic changes, allergic reactions, and seizures

-chlorpromazine and thioridazine and atypical antipsychotics clozapine, risperidone, olanzapine, and quetiapine antipsychotics most likely to cause orthostatic hypotension

-a/w **increased risk of sudden cardiac death**; **thioridazine** appears to carry highest risk of sudden unexplained death; risperidone prolongs QTc interval but has no effect on QT dispersion

Antiretroviral drugs, hepatotoxicity

-antiretroviral related liver injury (ARLI) is a **common cause** of **morbidity**, **mortality** and **tx discontinuation** in HIV-infected patients

-*every* licensed antiretroviral medication has been **a/w liver enzyme** *elevations*; some may cause liver injury more frequently than others

-several major mechanisms of ARLI include metabolic host mediated injury, hypersensitivity reactions, mitochondrial toxicity and immune phenomena

Antisocial Personality Disorder, alcohol abuse and dependence

-epidemiologic studies, *association* **b/w ASPD** and **alcohol abuse** and **dependence**

-Epidemiologic Catchment Area Survey, individuals meeting DSM criteria for **ASPD** were **21 times** *more likely* to develop **alcohol abuse and dependence** at some point during their lives

-study found that people w/ **ASPD** *before* **developing drinking problems** consumed **significantly more drinks per day**; experienced **significantly more alcohol-related problems** compared w/ people who did not meet criteria for ASPD

Anxiety Disorder, differential diagnosis

-**organic causes** *must* be **considered first** w/ *any* **acute change** in **mental status** or **sudden-onset change** in **behavior** in a previously well individual

-especially when **signs and sxs overlap w/ life-threatening condition** and when psychiatric syndrome being considered occurs outside of usual age window of presentation

-initial presentation w/ dyspnea, tachycardia, diaphoresis, chest pain, and light-headedness **should receive thorough medical evaluation** *before* being assigned dx of panic d/o

-should r/o unstable angina and MI, hypoglycemia, anemia, pulmonary embolism, asthma, obstructive pulmonary dz, GERD, irritable bowel dz, hyperparathyroidism, hyperthyroidism, pheochromocytoma, Huntington's dz, Parkinson's dz, seizure d/o, and autoimmune disorders, such as systemic lupus erythematosus

-use of benzodiazepine may be helpful to make patient more comfortable, but care should be taken not to mask sxs of more serious underlying condition

Aphasia

-disorder of verbal or written language rather than simply speech production

-almost always results results from **discrete lesions** in the **dominant cerebral hemisphere's perisylvian language arc**

-aspects of aphasia may occasionally result from Alzheimer's dz and degenerative conditions

Apraxia

-**loss of the ability** to execute or carry out **learned purposeful movements**, despite having the physical ability and motivation to perform the movements

-it is a disorder of motor planning which may be acquired or developmental

-NOT caused by incoordination, sensory loss, or failure to comprehend simple commands

-types include: ideomotor, ideational, verbal, constructional, oculomotor, limb kinetic

Asperger Disorder, clinical description

-in distinction from autistic d/o, "clinically significant general delay in language" and "cognitive delay" are exclusionary criteria

-significant **impairments in social interaction** and restricted and repetitive interests and behaviors are hallmarks

-unusual communication is common; often characterized by **pedantic speech**, intense **preoccupations**, and **poor or nonexistent nonverbal communication**

-it is commonly held that individuals w/ Asperger's d/o are clumsy

Aspirin and Vascular dementia

-observational data *suggest* **low-dose aspirin** *may* be **a/w reduced risk** of **cognitive decline and dementia**

-mechanism w/ Alzheimer's dz is uncertain

-low-dose aspirin reduces risk of stroke and this probably reduces risk of cognitive decline secondarily

-prospective randomized trials are needed to confirm whether aspirin can prevent cognitive decline

Astasia abasia

-**inability to stand or walk** in a normal manner

-**normal leg movements can be performed** in a sitting or lying down position

Astereognosis

-a variety of cortical sensory loss

-**inability** to **identify objects by touch**

-seen w/ lesions of the **contralateral parietal lobe**

Athetosis

-**involuntary** movement disorder

-usually results from **basal ganglia damage** from perinatal jaundice, anoxia, or prematurity

-characterized by **slow writhing, sinuous movement** of the arms or legs

-more pronounced in the distal part of the limbs

Atomoxetine, adolescents with ADHD and substance use disorder

-adolescents **presenting for substance use disorder** (SUD) tx have ***increased*** **rates of ADHD**, ranging from **30-50%**

-co-occurring ADHD is a/w **more severe substance use** and **worse substance use d/o outcomes**

-atomoxetine is **typically used to tx ADHD** in adolescents **w/ substance use d/o** because of its limited abuse potential

Attention-Deficit Hyperactivity Disorder, comorbidity

-individuals w/ADHD have poorer academic performance and **higher rates of Learning Disorders** than other children

-**inattentive** subtype may have more **anxiety and somatic complaints** than those w/combined or hyperactive–impulsive type; they have higher rates of Learning Disorders as well

Attention-Deficit Hyperactivity Disorder, comorbid depression

-comorbid conditions *should be considered* simultaneously; better understand sxs and optimal tx

-depressed patients demonstrate diminished concentration; w/ bipolar d/o often manifest psychomotor agitation and distractibility; *may be difficult to differentiate sxs* from cardinal sxs of ADHD

-long-term follow-up studies have demonstrated that individuals w/ **ADHD and comorbid disorders** have **poorer prognoses** and **greater hospitalization rates** than ADHD alone; ADHD and/or comorbid condition often persists for several years

-overlap b/w depression and ADHD is well recognized; children and adults referred for ADHD demonstrate higher than chance incidence of depression, individuals referred for depression show elevated rates of ADHD

-**depressed children** tend to present w/ **irritability, negativism, social withdrawal, school dysfunction,** and **somatic d/o**

-family studies suggest some genetic link b/w depression and ADHD, rates of ADHD among relatives of children w/ ADHD w/ or w/o depression were significantly higher than among relatives of controls

-stimulants do NOT significantly improve depression; tx for mood d/o are generally not helpful for ADHD

-in presence of a comorbid mood d/o, stimulants are less effective for ADHD; nonstimulant tx that is noradrenergic but not serotonergic are effective for ADHD; serotonergic antidepressants are effective for juvenile depression but not for ADHD

-**buproprion** (both noradrenergic and dopaminergic) shown to be efficacious for **adolescents w/ comorbid ADHD and depression**

Attention-Deficit Hyperactivity Disorder, course and prognosis

-course is variable; **~50%** of cases have sxs **persist into adolescence or adulthood**

-hyperactivity may disappear in some cases but decreased attention span and impulse-control problems persist

-overactivity is usually first symptom to remit; distractibility is last

-ADHD does NOT usually remit during middle childhood

-persistence is **predicted by family hx** of ADHD, **negative life events**, and **comorbidity** w/conduct sxs, depression, and anxiety d/o

-**remission** is unlikely before 12 yrs; **usually occurs b/w ages 12-20 yrs**

-most patients w/ ADHD have partial remission and are vulnerable to **antisocial behavior**, **substance use d/o**, and **mood d/o**

-**learning problems** often continue throughout life; **~40-50%** of cases have sxs persist into adulthood

-**adults** w/ ADHD *may* **show diminished hyperactivity**, but remain impulsive and accident-prone

-educational attainments as a group are lower than those w/o ADHD; early employment hx do not differ from those w/similar education

-children w/ sxs persisting into adolescence are at risk for developing conduct d/o

-children w/ both ADHD and conduct d/o are also at risk for developing a substance-related d/o; appears to be related to presence of conduct d/o rather than ADHD alone

-Most children w/ ADHD have some social difficulties; significantly higher rates of comorbid psychiatric disorders and experience more problems w/ behavior in school as well as w/ peers and family

Attunement

-Daniel **Stern** (1985) looked at developmental research and issues from a psychoanalytic perspective

-**affect attunement** is the ability to **know what the other person is experiencing subjectively**; not only emphatic understanding but also the **basis for early meaningful communication** and, most importantly, provides a **way for mutual appreciation of the other's mental state**

-highly attuned mothers foster **infant progression from being skilled dyadic partners to being skilled triadic partners**, who communicate readily about shared experiences in the world

-from an early age, Stern suggests that the child has the capacity to integrate different sensory information about an object in the world, and play an active role in their relationships w/ others

-children are gradually organizing and ordering them

-relationships to others are vital both for a sense of self and a sense of other as a separate other person in his or her own right

-affect attunement means a sharing or alignment of internal states in the domain of intersubjective relatedness

-attunement relates to the a) intensity b) timing and c) shape of a behavior; an example would be a mother responding w/ a sound and/or movement to her 9 month old child that corresponds equally to duration and amplitude of the child's cooing

Autism spectrum disorder, pharmacological treatment
Atypical antipsychotics

-**risperidone**; *only* atypical antipsychotic studied using randomized, double-blind methods and large number of patients, Research Units on Pediatric Psychopharmacology (RUPP) Autism Network

-tx w/ risperidone (dosage range, 0.5-3.5 mg/day) resulted in 56.9% reduction in irritability scores, compared to 14.1% decrease in placebo group

-improvements noted in stereotypic behavior and hyperactivity

-2/3 of children w/ positive response to risperidone at 8 weeks, benefit was maintained at 6 mos

-social isolation and interest in communicating w/ others did not differ significantly b/w tx and placebo

-similar results in children w/ subaverage intelligence and no autism; sxs of conduct problems, irritability, and hyperactivity responded to risperidone

Selective Serotonin Reuptake Inhibitors

-demonstrated effectiveness in *reducing* **aggression**, **irritability**, **stereotypies**, and other **disruptive behaviors**, no SSRI has been shown to be superior to another

-**no** SSRI has been shown to improve specific **social communication sxs**

Aversive conditioning, or punishment
-procedure in which **punishment** or **aversive stimulus** is used to **reduce frequency** of a target behavior

Avoidant Personality Disorder, differential diagnosis
-schizoid PD also involves social isolation, but schizoid person does NOT desire relationships

-avoidant person **desires relationships** but avoids them because of anxiety and fears of humiliation and rejection

-avoidant PD is characterized by **avoidance of situations and relationships** involving *possible* **rejection**, **disappointment**, **ridicule**, or **shame**

-Axis I social phobia usually consists of specific fears related to social performance (e.g., fear of saying something inappropriate or of being unable to answer questions in front of other people)

B

Bell palsy, clinical features

-**most common** cause of **unilateral facial paralysis**, also known as idiopathic facial paralysis

- ~60-75% of cases w/ acute unilateral facial paralysis

-dx of exclusion (exclude recent or past trauma), clinical features may help distinguish it from other causes of facial paralysis

-dx made on basis of thorough hx and examination, sxs include:

Acute onset of **unilateral upper and lower facial paralysis** (over 48-hrs)

Posterior auricular pain, occurs in 1/2

Decreased **tearing**, occurs in 1/6

Hyperacusis, occurs in 1/3 d/t stapedius muscle weakness

Taste disturbances

-paralysis must include forehead and lower aspect of face

-may report **inability to close eye or smile** on affected side

-may report *increased* **saliva** on side of the paralysis

-central lesion or cause should be suspected, supranuclear; if paralysis involves only lower portion of face

-stroke or intracerebral lesion; if contralateral weakness or diplopia in conjunction w/ supranuclear facial palsy

-many report numbness on side of paralysis, possibly trigeminal nerve involvement; others suggest d/t lack of mobility of facial muscles, not lack of sensation

-gradual onset of facial paralysis, weakness of contralateral side, or hx of trauma or infection strongly suggest other causes

-GBS, Lyme dz (5-10% peripheral seventh nerve palsy), and meningitis should be considered in bilateral facial palsy

-tumor of the seventh nerve or parotid gland should be suspected in recurrent ipsilateral facial paralysis

-Ramsay Hunt syndrome should be considered w/ sudden onset of hearing loss and severe pain w/ onset of facial paralysis

Benzodiazepine, seizure risk in alcohol detoxification

-typical outpatient regimen requires patient to attend the clinic daily for 5-10 days to receive clinical evaluations, multiple vitamins, and gradually decreasing benzodiazepine pharmacotherapy

-typical medication dosing regimen involves giving enough benzodiazepine on first day of tx to relieve withdrawal sxs

-dose should be adjusted if withdrawal sxs increase or if patient complains of excessive sedation

-over next 5-7 days, dose of benzodiazepine is tapered to zero

-most clinicians use longer-acting benzodiazepines such as clonazepam, chlordiazepoxide, or diazepam; **shorter-acting** benzodiazepines increase likelihood of **grand mal seizures**

-usual starting dose of medication on first day is 25-50 mg of chlordiazepoxide (max 300 mg daily) or 10 mg of diazepam given every 6 hours; **chlordiazepoxide** and longer acting benzodiazepines ***should* be avoided** in individuals **w/ liver dz** (hepatitis, cirrhosis, etc.)

-in outpatient setting, **oxazepam** may be particularly useful because it is **a/w less abuse** and **does NOT require hepatic biotransformation**, an important consideration for alcoholics w/ liver dz

Bereavement, diagnostic criteria

-focus of clinical attention is **reaction to death of loved one**

-some present w/ sxs characteristic of Major Depressive Episode

-individual typically regards depressed mood as normal; may seek professional help for relief of insomnia or anorexia

-duration and expression of bereavement vary considerably among different cultures

-dx of MDD is generally not given unless sxs are still present 2 months after the loss

-presence of certain sxs **NOT** characteristic of normal grief reaction may *differentiate* bereavement from a **Major Depressive Episode**

1) **guilt** about things *other than* **actions taken or not taken** by survivor at time of death

2) **thoughts of death** *other than* the survivor feeling that he or she **would be better off dead** or **should have died** w/ deceased person

3) **morbid preoccupation** w/ **worthlessness**

4) *marked* **psychomotor retardation**

5) *prolonged* and *marked* **functional impairment**

6) **hallucinatory** experiences *other than* thinking that he or she hears the voice of, or transiently sees the image of, the deceased person

Beta-adrenergic receptor antagonists, treatment for akathisia

-historically, reported to be effective for tx of restless legs syndrome, or Ekbom's syndrome (1965), which resembles physical movements of akathisia

-later, reported to be effective in tx of **neuroleptic-induced akathisia**

-in **CNS**, produce **fatigue, sleep disturbance** (insomnia and nightmares), and CNS **depression**

-all beta-blockers undergo metabolism in liver

-propranolol and metoprolol undergo significant first-pass effect, w/ bioavailability as low as 25%

-large interindividual variation (as much as 20-fold) leads to wide variation in clinically therapeutic doses

-exact **mechanism of action** of beta-blockers in the **tx of EPS** is **unclear**

-existence of a **noradrenergic pathway** from **locus coeruleus** *to* **limbic system** has been proposed as modulator involved in sxs of **TD, akathisia**, and **tremor**

-lipid solubility and corresponding ability to enter CNS are most important factors determining efficacy of a beta-blocker in tx of akathisia

-indicated for familial essential tremor; **no FDA-approved indications** for tx of any type of **EPS**

-both nonselective (beta1 and beta2 antagonism) and selective (beta1 antagonism) beta-blockers have been reported to be efficacious in tx of akathisia

-maximum benefit for propranolol occurred at 5 days; betaxolol may be beta-blocker of choice in patients w/ lung dz and smokers because of its beta1 selectivity at lower dosages (5-10 mg/day)

Borderline Personality Disorder, associated features and disorders
-may have a **pattern of undermining themselves** at the moment a goal is about to be realized (school, therapy, relationships)

-Some develop **psychotic-like sxs** (e.g., hallucinations, body-image distortions, ideas of reference, and hypnagogic phenomena) **during times of stress**

-*may* feel ***more* secure w/ transitional objects** (i.e., a pet or inanimate possession) *than* in interpersonal relationships

-premature death from **suicide** may occur; especially co-occurring Mood D/O or Substance-Related D/O

-physical handicaps may result from **self-inflicted abuse** behaviors or *failed* **suicide attempts**

-recurrent job losses, interrupted education, and broken marriages are common

-physical and sexual **abuse**, **neglect**, hostile **conflict**, and *early* **parental loss** or **separation** is more common in childhood hx

-common **co-occurring Axis I** disorders include Mood D/O, Substance-Related D/O, Eating D/O (notably Bulimia), PTSD, and ADHD

-frequently co-occurs w/ other Personality Disorders

Borderline Personality Disorder, etiology
-psychoanalytic theories emphasized **importance of early parent-child relationships** (Johnson et al. 2005a)

1) **maternal mismanagement of 2- to 3-year-old child's efforts** to become **autonomous** (Masterson 1972)

2) exaggerated **maternal frustration** that **aggravates child's anger** (Kernberg 1975)

3)   **inattention** to **child's emotions and attitudes** (Adler 1985)

-**lack of reliably involved attachment to caretakers during development** is a source of borderline patients' inability to maintain stable senses of themselves or of others w/o ongoing contact (**fail to achieve object constancy**; lack of stable introjects) (Gunderson 1996)

-Zanarini and Frankenburg (1997) proposed a tripartite causative model of BPD consisting of a traumatic childhood, a vulnerable temperament, and triggering events

-Linehan's **biosocial theory** suggests biological disposition toward **emotional vulnerability**, exposure to **invalidating environments**, and deficits in **emotion-regulation skills** (Linehan 1993)

-Joyce et al. (2003) proposed distinctive combination of risk factors consisting of a temperament characterized by high novelty seeking and high harm avoidance, childhood abuse and/or neglect, and childhood or adolescent psychopathology in the affective, conduct, and substance abuse domains

-Posner et al. (2003) included a combination of high negative emotionality and a deficit in an executive attentional control network

-Siever and Davis (1991) posited fundamental dimensions of affective instability and impulsive aggression underlying BPD

-Livesley et al. 1993) found heritability of about 50% for borderline traits; affective lability and insecure attachment, as well as broader domains of emotional dysregulation and dissocial behavior (Livesley et al. 1998)

-evidence of serotonergic dysfunction in borderline trait of impulsivity

-structural and functional neuroimaging studies have shown **reductions in frontal and orbitofrontal lobe volumes, altered metabolism in prefrontal brain regions**, and **failure of activation of these brain regions under stress**

-other studies have shown **hyperactivity of the amygdala**, which also plays a central role in emotion regulation

-perform poorly in multiple neurocognitive domains, particularly on **functions *lateralized* to right hemisphere**

Borderline Personality Disorder, increase risk of suicide attempt/completion
-**most concerning** is *current* or *past* **substance use d/o**; a/w increased lifetime suicide attempts

-can **disinhibit** individuals who may be ambivalent about suicide, leading to more lethal attempts

-can **impair judgment** so that suicidal actions instigated w/ a low level of intent can result in lethal consequences

-substance use disorders *may* **be linked** to the **trait of impulsivity**; considered a suicide risk factor even after substance abuse or MDD is controlled

-suicide attempters w/ co-occurring Borderline PD and MDD have **more** lifetime suicide **attempts**; make **first attempt at a younger age**; report **more interpersonal triggers**; higher levels of lifetime **aggressive behaviors**, **hostility**, and **impulsivity** compared w/ depressed attempters w/o Borderline PD

-*current* **severity of MDD** is a/w increased risk for a greater number of suicide attempts that are more lethal in Borderline PD

Breathing-Related Sleep Disorder

-essential feature is **sleep disruption**, leading to **excessive sleepiness** or, less commonly, to insomnia, that is judged to be d/t abnormalities of ventilation during sleep (e.g., sleep apnea or central alveolar hypoventilation)

-must not be better accounted for by mental disorder and is not d/t direct physiological effects of substance (including medication) or a general medical condition that produces sleep sxs through mechanism other than abnormal breathing

-excessive sleepiness is most common presenting complaint of individuals w/Breathing-Related Sleep D/O (BRSD)

-sleepiness results from **frequent arousals during nocturnal sleep** as individual attempts to breathe normally

-sleepiness is most evident in relaxing situations, such as reading or watching TV

-**inability to control sleepiness** can be evident in boring meetings or while attending movies, theater, or concerts

-when sleepiness is **extreme**, *may* **fall asleep while actively conversing, eating, walking**, or **driving**

-naps tend to be unrefreshing and may be accompanied by dull headache on awakening

-impact of the sleepiness may be minimized and individual may express pride about being able to sleep anywhere at any time

-insomnia, frequent awakenings, or unrefreshing sleep are less frequent than daytime sleepiness as presenting complaint

-abnormal respiratory events during sleep include apneas (episodes of breathing cessation), hypopneas (abnormally slow or shallow respiration), and hypoventilation (abnormal blood oxygen and carbon dioxide levels)

-3 forms of BRSD: **obstructive sleep apnea syndrome** (most common), central sleep apnea syndrome, and central alveolar hypoventilation syndrome

-older term, Pickwickian syndrome, has been used to describe obese individuals w/combination of OSA and waking hypoventilation

Bromocriptine, Restless Leg Syndrome

-term restless legs syndrome (RLS) used initially in mid-1940s by Swedish neurologist Karl A. Ekbom to describe a disorder characterized by **sensory sxs**, including unpleasant **aching** and **crawling feelings** in **calves and thighs**, and **motor disturbances of limbs**, mainly during **rest** and at **bedtime**

- ~5-15% of general population, w/ **female-to-male ratio of 2:1**

-may report sensations as an almost **irresistible urge to move legs (walking provides temporary relief)**, which are **not painful** but distinctly bothersome; can lead to significant physical and emotional disability

-sensations usually are worse during inactivity and often **interfere w/ sleep**, leading to walking discomfort, chronic sleep deprivation, and stress

-pathogenesis of RLS is unclear; most widely accepted mechanism involves genetic component along w/ **abnormalities** in **central, subcortical dopamine pathways** and **impaired iron homeostasis**

-sxs are reactivated when centrally acting dopamine receptor antagonists are administered to pts w/ syndrome

-results of SPECT imaging have suggested deficiency of dopamine D2 receptors

-abnormalities of iron homeostasis have also been implicated, based on CSF iron profile measures

-All patients w/ low iron levels (ferritin <50 ng/mL) should receive supplemental iron therapy; ferrous sulfate 325 mg may be given w/ 250 mg of vitamin C; absorption is increased by taking this on empty stomach and waiting 60 min before eating

-**dopaminergic agents**; may improve sensory sxs a/w RLS

-agents like **pramipexole**, **ropinirole**, and **bromocriptine** are less likely than combination drug levodopa/carbidopa to produce augmentation or rebound; can be used alone or along w/ levodopa

-*adverse effects* of dopamine agonists include **nausea**, **light-headedness**, **drowsiness**, and **postural hypotension**

-levodopa/carbidopa is generally reserved for patients w/ infrequent sxs because of problems w/ augmentation and rebound

Bulimia Nervosa, medical complications
Binge eating

-acute dilatation of stomach—shock

Self-induced vomiting

-esophageal tears—shock; dehydration

-metabolic alkalosis—hypochloremia, hypokalemia, weakness, lethargy

-cardiac arrhythmias—cardiac arrest

-erosion of dental enamel—caries, exposure of pulp

Parotid gland enlargement (self induced vomiting or excessive gum chewing)

-elevated serum amylase

Ipecac use

-hypotension, tachycardia, electrocardiographic abnormalities, elevated liver enzymes

Buprenorphine, sublingual administration
-**mixed agonist-antagonist**, approved by FDA in 2002 as an alternative to methadone for maintenance tx of opiate addiction

-allowed possibility of office-based tx outside highly regulated methadone clinics

-available as schedule III drug (methadone is schedule II)

-studies support outpatient-based buprenorphine therapy is highly effective in reducing relapse and enhancing adherence in 12-step programs and may be safer than methadone tx

-usual dosage 6-20 mg/day, w/ target dosage of around 16 mg/day

-taken **sublingually** to **avoid excessive drug destruction in the liver**, which occurs if drug is taken as ordinary pill and swallowed

-sublingual form, most widely used analgesic in many European countries

-well tolerated and elicit very mild dependence and withdrawal sxs, even after prolonged high-dose administration

-can substitute for other opiates and can block opiate-induced euphoria

-decreases illicit drug use, as measured by urine screens, as effectively as methadone (not completely, but substantially)

-studies of buprenorphine in opiate withdrawal suggest it is equivalent in efficacy to methadone and superior to other drugs, such as clonidine

-withdrawing patients from maintenance buprenorphine is much easier than withdrawing from methadone

C

Caffeine
-**most commonly** used **mood-altering drug** in the world

-found in numerous plants; most widely consumed being coffee, tea, cola nut, cocao pod, guarana, and maté

-estimated that **80-90% of adults and children** in U.S. habitually consume caffeine

- ~15% of general population report having stopped caffeine use completely, citing concern about health and unpleasant side effects

Capgras syndrome
-**unspecified type of delusion**; reserved for cases in which predominant delusion cannot be subtyped w/in jealous, persecutory, erotomanic, grandiose, somatic

-named for French psychiatrist who described *illusion des sosies*, or the **illusion of doubles**

-delusion is belief that a **familiar person has been replaced by an impostor**

-variants include the delusion that **persecutors or familiar persons can assume the guise of strangers (Frégoli's** phenomenon) and the very rare delusion that **familiar persons can change themselves into other persons at will (intermetamorphosis)**

-each disorder is not only rare but may be a/w schizophrenia, dementia, epilepsy, and other organic disorders, including CNS lesions, vitamin B12 deficiency, hepatic encephalopathy, diabetes, and hypothyroidism

-reported cases have been predominantly in women, have had associated paranoid features, and have included feelings of depersonalization or derealization

-delusion may be short lived, recurrent, or persistent

-unclear whether delusional d/o can appear w/ such a delusion; Frégoli and intermetamorphosis delusions have bizarre content and are unlikely, but the delusion in Capgras syndrome is a possible candidate for delusional d/o

-role of hallucination or perceptual disturbance in this condition needs to be explicated; cases have appeared after sudden brain damage

Carbamazepine, interaction w/ haloperidol

-carbamazepine is an **inducer** of CYP3A4 isoenzyme

-concomitant use w/ some antipsychotic agents (e.g., aripiprazole, clozapine, **haloperidol**, risperidone, ziprasidone) has been shown, or would be expected, to **decrease plasma concentrations of the antipsychotic agent**

-reductions in antipsychotic efficacy w/ reemergence of psychotic sxs has occurred in some, but not all

-if carbamazepine tx is added in patients receiving aripiprazole; dosage of aripiprazole should be doubled and additional increases in aripiprazole dosage should be made based on clinical evaluation

-if carbamazepine is withdrawn from combination therapy w/ aripiprazole, dosage of aripiprazole should be reduced accordingly

-patients receiving **carbamazepine and haloperidol concomitantly** should be **monitored carefully for loss of antipsychotic control** and, if an interaction is suspected, haloperidol dosage adjusted accordingly

-possibility that **haloperidol toxicity** *may* occur following **discontinuance of carbamazepine** also should be considered

Carbon monoxide poisoning, Globus palladus

-carbon monoxide may cause brain lipid peroxidation and leukocyte-mediated inflammatory changes

-severe intoxication; CNS pathology may include white matter demyelination leading to edema and focal areas of necrosis, typically of **bilateral globus pallidus**; most likely **secondary to hypoperfusion and hypoxia** since affected tissues are considered watershed areas w/ relatively low oxygen demand

-**CT** may be positive **w/in 24 hrs, MRI sooner**

-characteristic finding is bilateral, **symmetric low attenuation lesions in globus palladus**

-may also demonstrate low density lesions in cerebral and cerebellar white matter w/ sparing of subcortical fibers

-positive CT findings herald long-term neurologic complications, may occasionally follow period of lucidity lasting days to weeks

-MRI, produces low or high signal intensity lesions on T1, high intensity signal on T2 in globus pallidus

-globus pallidus lesions on imaging findings **may also be seen w/ hypoxic-anoxic injuries**, may involve caudate nucleus and other central gray nuclei; Wilson's dz may have hypodensities in basal ganglia and thalami; cyanide can produce globus pallidus infarctions and early diffuse cerebral edema

-tx'd w/ 100% oxygen; dz process may be inhibited by hyperbaric oxygen therapy, remains controversial

Case-control study

-type of **retrospective**, **epidemiological** study design

-appropriate when **incidence of dz is low**

-individuals **w/ dz** are **matched** w/individuals who **do not have dz**, or controls

-**compares** groups of people **based on dz**; information is collected **retrospectively** w/ regards to **exposure**

-examines **whether exposure occurred more frequently** *or* **less frequently** in individuals **w/ dz vs. individuals w/o dz** (controls)

-**retrospective**, **non-randomized** nature *limits* the strength of their conclusions

-**less expensive** and generally is **less time-consuming** than cohort studies and randomized controlled trials

Catatonic type, schizophrenia

-common several decades ago, has become rare in Europe and North America

-classic feature is a marked disturbance in motor function; may involve stupor, negativism, rigidity, excitement, or posturing

-may show rapid alteration b/w extremes of excitement and stupor

-associated features include stereotypies, mannerisms, and waxy flexibility

-mutism is particularly common

-during catatonic excitement, patients need careful supervision to prevent them from hurting themselves or others

-medical care may be needed because of malnutrition, exhaustion, hyperpyrexia, or self-inflicted injury

-clinical picture is dominated by **at least 2 of following**:

Motoric immobility, evidenced by catalepsy (including waxy flexibility) or **stupor**

Excessive motor activity (**purposeless** and not influenced by external stimuli)

Extreme negativism (apparently motiveless resistance to all instructions or maintenance of rigid posture against attempts to be moved) or **mutism**

Peculiarities of voluntary movement, posturing (voluntary assumption of inappropriate or **bizarre postures**), **stereotyped movements**, prominent mannerisms, or prominent grimacing

Echolalia or **echopraxia**

Caudate nucleus, Obsessive-Compulsive Disorder

-theorized that caudate nucleus **may be dysfunctional in OCD**

-inappropriately *increased* **activity in head of caudate nucleus** *inhibits* **globus pallidus fibers** that ordinarily dampen thalamic activity; *increase* **in thalamic activity** produces *increased* **activity in orbitofrontal cortex**, which produces *increased* **activity in the head of the caudate** through the cingulate gyrus

-may be **unable to properly regulate transmission** of information regarding **worrying events or ideas** b/w **thalamus and orbitofrontal cortex**

-**PET** scan studies have found *increased* metabolism in **orbital frontal cortex, cingulate gyrus**, and **caudate**, w/ decreases following successful tx

-meta-analyses of voxel-based morphometry studies comparing individuals w/ OCD and healthy controls find that individuals w/ OCD have increased grey matter volumes in bilateral lenticular nuclei extending to the caudate nuclei

Cerebellar tremor

-**slow, broad tremor** of **extremities** that **occurs at the end of a purposeful movement**, such as trying to press a button or touching a finger to the tip of one's nose

-frequency ~**3 Hz**, **irregular amplitude**

-caused by **lesions** in, or **damage** to, **cerebellum** resulting from stroke, tumor, or dz such as multiple sclerosis or some inherited degenerative disorder

-can also result from chronic alcoholism or overuse of some medicines

-a lesion on one side of the brain **produces a tremor in that *same* side of the body** that **worsens w/ directed movement**

-cerebellar damage can also produce a "wing-beating" type of tremor called rubral or Holmes' tremor, which is a combination of rest, action, and postural tremors

-tremor is often most prominent when affected person is active or is maintaining a particular posture

-may be accompanied by dysarthria (speech problems), nystagmus (rapid, involuntary rolling of the eyes), gait problems, and postural tremor of the trunk and neck

-typically does NOT respond to medical tx; patients w/rubral tremor may receive some relief using levodopa or anticholinergic drugs

Child Behavior Checklist (CBCL)

-parent and teacher versions developed to cover **broad range of psychiatric sxs**, as well as several positive attributes related to **academic** and **social competence**

-presents items related to mood, frustration tolerance, hyperactivity, oppositional behavior, anxiety, and various other behaviors

-parent version consists of 118 items to be rated 0 (not true), 1 (sometimes true), or 2 (very true)

-teacher version is similar, but w/o items referring to home life

-**normative data** from normal children of **3 different age groups** (4-5 yrs, 6-11 yrs, and 12-16 yrs)

-**identifies specific problem areas** that might otherwise be overlooked; may point out areas in which child's behavior **deviates from normal children of *same* age group**

-**NOT** used specifically **to make diagnoses**

-revised CBCL; 150 items that cover variety of childhood behavioral and emotional sxs; discriminates b/w clinic-referred and nonreferred children

Childhood-onset schizophrenia

-rare and severe form of schizophrenia characterized by an onset of psychotic sxs by **age 12 yrs**

-**onset** is frequently **insidious**; may take months or years to meet all diagnostic criteria for schizophrenia

-thought to occur in affected individuals w/increased heritable etiology

-high rates of premorbid developmental abnormalities

-imaging studies; suggest decreased anterior cingulated gyrus (ACG) volumes w/age, unlike controls, and an absence of the normal decreased left to right ACG volume asymmetry

-hypothesized to be related to abnormal neurodevelopment influencing attention and emotion regulation

-frequency reported to be <1 in 10,000 children

-*extremely* **high rates of comorbid psychiatric disorders** are seen, including ADHD, depressive disorders, and separation anxiety disorder

Circumstantiality

-disturbance in **associative thought** and **speech processes**

-patient **lacks goal directedness** and **digresses** into **unnecessary details** and **inappropriate thoughts** before communicating the central idea

-observed during mental status examination in schizophrenia, obsessional disturbances, and certain cases of dementia

Clang association

-type of **disorganization** of the form or **thought process** as evident in language output

-association or speech **directed by the sound of a word** rather than by its meaning

-stringing together **words w/ no logical connection** based on **phonetic similarities**; e.g., hat, cat, sat, fat

-punning and rhyming may dominate verbal behavior

-seen most frequently in schizophrenia or mania

Classic conditioning

-**association** of a **neutral stimulus w/ unconditioned stimulus**

-**neutral stimulus** comes to elicit a **response similar** to **unconditioned stimulus**

Clonidine, opioid detoxification

-**alpha$_2$-adrenergic agonist** drug clonidine has been used (**considered standard tx**) to facilitate **opioid withdrawal in both inpatient and outpatient settings**

-0.6-2.0 mg/day **reduces many autonomic components of opioid withdrawal** syndrome; craving, lethargy, insomnia, restlessness, and muscle aches are NOT well suppressed

-believed to exert its **ameliorative actions** by **binding to alpha$_2$**-autoreceptors in **brain** (e.g., **locus coeruleus) and spinal cord**

-*both* opioids and clonidine can **suppress activity of locus coeruleus**, which is hyperactive during opioid withdrawal

-inpatients stabilized at 50 mg/day or less of methadone can be switched abruptly to clonidine

-dosages reaching 2.5 mg/day during precipitated withdrawal and antagonist induction have been used, w/ careful monitoring of HR and BP to minimize risk of significant hypotension and/or syncope; sedation and hypotension are major side effects

-used for outpatient detoxification from either heroin or methadone maintenance

-patients maintained on 20 mg/day or less of methadone are about as successful after abrupt substitution of clonidine as after reduction of methadone by 1 mg/day

-has NOT been given official FDA approval for use in controlling withdrawal, but it has been used so widely now, both in U.S. and abroad, that it has become accepted as an alternative to gradual methadone reduction

-has mild analgesic effects; pain usually returns 24-48 hrs after last clonidine dose; if naltrexone is used, pain needs to be tx'd w/ nonopioid analgesics

Clozapine, prolactin levels
-first of the class of atypical antisychotic drugs

-landmark in tx of schizophrenia for several reasons: first medication shown to be **efficacious in o/w nonresponsive patients**; first agent to **significantly attenuate negative sxs** of schizophrenia, such as marked social withdrawal and apathy

-**rarely produces EPS**, and to date is the *only* antipsychotic drug *not* **a/w treatment-emergent TD**

-**chronic** administration of clozapine results in **selective inhibition of dopamine neurons** in **mesolimbic pathways** w/ *little* **functional effect** on **striatal dopamine tracts**

-**minimal** effects on **tuberoinfundibular** system; does **NOT** cause **hyperprolactinemia**

Clozapine, seizure risk dose-dependent
-a/w **dose-dependent risk** of **seizures**

-vast **majority** of clozapine-induced seizures are **tonic-clonic**, but myoclonic seizures also occur

- **< 300 mg/day** are a/w **1-3% risk** of seizures

-**300-600 mg/day** carry **2.7% risk**, and doses **> 600 mg/day** are a/w **4.4% risk**

-doses **> 600 mg/day** are **NOT recommended** unless patient's sxs have not responded at lower doses

-once a seizure has occurred, decision to continue clozapine requires clinical judgment

Clozapine, suicide risk in schizophrenia

-may be **preferred agent** for patients w/schizophrenia who are **at higher risk for suicide**

-large epidemiological studies have found mortality from suicide is reduced among individuals taking clozapine (Reid et al. 1998; Walker et al. 1997)

-*reduction* **in number of serious suicide attempts** as well as in expressed depression and hopelessness found in patients who were changed to clozapine (Meltzer and Okayli, 1995)

-most convincing study was comparison of clozapine and olanzapine in 980 patients w/schizophrenia who were considered at risk for suicide; clozapine was *more* **effective in** *reducing* **risk of suicide** (Meltzer 2002)

Clozapine, agranulocytosis

-**agranulocytosis** estimated to occur in **0.8% of patients** receiving clozapine during first year of tx; **peak incidence at 3 months**

-hematological monitoring has reduced agranulocytosis-related fatalities to extremely low levels

-dispensing of clozapine in U.S. is linked to **weekly** WBC counts **during first 6 months** and **biweekly** counts **thereafter**

-strict guidelines based on WBC and absolute neutrophil counts have been set:

Initial white blood cell (**WBC**) count *must* be **> 3,500/mm^3**, and absolute neutrophil count (**ANC**) *must* be **>2,000/mm^3**

Weekly WBC count and ANC are required for first 6 months of tx and for **4 weeks after discontinuation of clozapine**; after 6 months, monitoring is required every 2 weeks; and **after 12 months**, monitoring is *required* **every 4 weeks**

If WBC count is 2,000-3,000/mm^3 or **ANC is 1,000-1,500/mm^3**, **interrupt** therapy and **monitor for signs of infection**; perform WBC and differential counts **daily**; if no sxs of infection are seen, **if WBC count returns** to **> 3,000/mm^3**, and **if ANC is > 1,500/mm^3**, resume clozapine therapy w/ **twice-weekly WBC and differential counts** until total WBC count returns to more than 3,500/mm3 and ANC is > 2,000/mm3

If WBC count is **< 2,000/mm^3** or **ANC is < 1,000/mm^3**, **discontinue** clozapine and do **NOT rechallenge**; perform WBC and differential counts **daily** until WBC count is > 3,000/mm^3 and ANC is > 1,500/mm^3, then monitor twice weekly until WBC count returns to more than 3,500/mm^3 and ANC is greater than 2,000/mm^3, then monitor weekly for 4 weeks

Treat any infection w/ antibiotics; consider bone marrow aspiration to ascertain granulopoietic status; if granulopoiesis is deficient, consider protective isolation

-since implementation of Clozaril National Registry in U.S., rate of agranulocytosis has been ~0.38% on basis of data collected from FEB '90-DEC '94

-if agranulocytosis develops, **prompt consultation w/ hematologist** is indicated

-reverse isolation and prophylactic antibiotics may be used to prevent infection

-granulocyte colony-stimulating factors may be used to shorten duration and reduce morbidity of agranulocytosis

-although **lithium** *often* **causes leukocytosis**, it **does NOT** appear to **treat or prevent clozapine**-induced **agranulocytosis**

-once a patient has developed agranulocytosis while taking clozapine, he or she should NOT be rechallenged w/ clozapine

-clozapine is **contraindicated** in patients who have **myeloproliferative disorders** or who are **immunocompromised** as a result of diseases such as active tuberculosis or HIV infection because of their increased risk for agranulocytosis

-concomitant administration of medications that are **a/w bone marrow suppression**, such as **carbamazepine**, is also **contraindicated**

Clozapine, extrapyramidal side effects
-**EPS** are **uncommon w/any dose** of clozapine

-*some* patients experience **akathisia** or **hand tremors**

-risk for NMS exists; has been reported w/ individuals medicated w/ clozapine alone

Cognitive Development, 4 Stages
-developed by Jean **Piaget**

-emphasizes the way children **think** and **acquire knowledge**

-**4 major stages** leading to adult capacity for thought:

1. **sensorimotor (up to 2 yrs)**; acquire **control of motor functions** and idea of **object permanence**

2. **preoperational thought (2-7 yrs)**; **symbols** and **language** are used, ideas of imminent justice and **magical thinking** exist, child is **egocentric**

3. **concrete operations (7-11 yrs)**; egocentric thought is *replaced* by **operational thought, syllogistic reasoning** occurs, **conservation** and **reversibility** are understood

4. **formal operations (11 yrs to end of adolescence)**; which involves acquiring **deductive reasoning skills** and **abstract thinking** w/ use of **complex language**

Cognitive function with aging, speech and language
-**speech and language processing are largely intact** in older adults under normal conditions; **processing time** *may* be somewhat **slower** than in young adults

-evidence that discourse skills actually improve w/ age; usually have more extensive vocabularies

-may exhibit occasional word-finding difficulty, older adults easily able to provide circumlocutions to mask problem

-older people seem able to engage intact top-down processes to bolster deficiencies in bottom-up processing

-appear to retain good language skills well into older age

-deficits that occur under difficult processing conditions seem primarily attributable to sensory loss or working memory limitations, NOT to impairments in basic language capacities

Competence, Industry versus Inferiority (~5-13yrs)
-**onset of latency**, child **discovers pleasures of production**

-develops industry by learning new skills and takes pride in things made

-Erikson wrote in Childhood and Society that child's "ego boundaries include his tools and skills: the work principle teaches him the pleasure of work completion by steady attention and persevering diligence."

-across cultures; child receives systematic instruction and learns fundamentals of technology as they pertain to use of basic utensils and tools

-identify w/ their teachers and imagine themselves in various occupational roles

-child who is **unprepared** for this stage of psychosocial development, either through **insufficient resolution of previous stages** or by **current interference**, *may* develop a sense of **inferiority and inadequacy**

-society becomes crucially important in child's ability to overcome sense of inferiority and to achieve the virtue known as **competence**

-In Identity: Youth and Crisis, Erikson noted: "This is socially a most decisive stage since industry involves doing things beside and w/ others, a first sense of division of labor and of differential opportunity, that is, a sense of the technological ethos of a culture, develops at this time."

-pathological outcome of a poorly navigated stage of industry versus inferiority is less well defined than in previous stages

-may concern the emergence of a conformist immersion; creativity is stifled and identity is subsumed under the worker's role

Competency

-legally, **only competent** persons may give **informed consent**

-**ALL** individuals, including those dx'd w/ mental illness, are **legally presumed to be competent** to make all decisions (medical and mental health tx decisions) unless adjudicated incompetent or temporarily incapacitated because of medical emergency

-NOT a global concept but is measured **in terms of specific decisions or abilities**: competence to enter into contracts, make medical decisions, execute a will, participate in studies or experimentation, manage finances, vote, and other individual tasks or projects

-different activities require different standards of competence; recognized by both clinicians and courts; person may be competent for decision making about medical tx, but not about management of financial affairs

-NO single accepted test for competence for individual and specific tasks

-clinically useful to distinguish terms incompetence and incapacity; *incompetence* refers to a **court adjudication**, whereas *incapacity* indicates **functional inability** as determined by a clinician

-incapacity does not prevent tx; it merely requires clinician to obtain substitute consent or an exception to requirement of informed consent

Competency to Stand Trial

-legal standard for **assessing pretrial competency** was established by U.S. Supreme Court in ***Dusky v. United States 1960***

-to be competent to make decisions during pretrial process, at trial, and during an appeal, the court required that defendant have "sufficient present ability to consult w/ his lawyer w/ a reasonable degree of rational understanding" and "has a rational as well as factual understanding of the proceedings against him" *Dusky v. United States 1960*

-the Dusky test does NOT require absence of understanding resulting from the presence of a mental dz or defect (although it is typical)

-defendant may be found incompetent to stand trial even if he or she does not have a mental dz or defect (physical illness that affects cognition)

-*most* impairment implicated in competency examinations is **functional rather than organic**

-in *Wilson v. United States 1968*, permanent retrograde amnesia from injury after robbery; criteria that court established in determining defendant's competency to stand trial: extent to which amnesia affected defendant's ability to consult w/ and assist his lawyer; extent to which amnesia affected defendant's ability to testify in his own behalf

-actual *functional* **mental capability to meet minimal standard of trial competency**, and **NOT severity** of deficits determines whether individual is cognitively capable to be tried; legal criteria, NOT medical or psychiatric dx, that govern competency

-Interdisciplinary Fitness Interview, designed for use by lawyers and MH professionals (Schreiber et al. 1987), provides detailed examination of psychopathology and legal knowledge using explicit scales for rating each response to competency evaluation; *should* **avoid detailed hx of defendant's past offenses during eval**

-defendant's **impairment in *one* particular function does *not* automatically render him or her incompetent**; a defendant manifesting certain deficits because of damage to parietal lobe does not necessarily mean that he or she lacks requisite cognitive ability to aid in his or her own defense at trial (Tranel 1992)

-ultimate determination of incompetency is for the court to decide *United States v. David 1975*; impairment must be considered in context of particular case or proceeding

-mental impairment that may render an individual incompetent to stand trial in a complicated tax fraud case might not for a misdemeanor trial

-psychiatrists and psychologists who testify as expert witnesses regarding effect of psychiatric problems on defendant's competency to stand trial are **most effective if their findings are framed** according to the *degree* **to which the defendant is** *cognitively capable* **of meeting the standards** enunciated in Dusky

Condensation

-mechanism by which **several unconscious wishes**, **impulses**, or **attitudes** can be **combined into a single image** in manifest **dream content**; monster in child's dream representing dreamer's father, mother, or even the child's own primitive hostile impulses

-converse of condensation can also occur; irradiation or diffusion of a single latent wish or impulse that is distributed through multiple representations in manifest dream content

-combination of mechanisms of condensation and diffusion provides the dreamer w/ highly flexible and economic device for facilitating, compressing, and diffusing or expanding manifest dream content, which is derived from latent or unconscious wishes and impulses

Conduction aphasia

-occurs in **left arcuate fasciculus** region

-gives *fluent* spontaneous **speech**, *good* auditory **comprehension**, and **poor repetition and naming**

Confidentiality

-essential for effective tx, particularly psychotherapy

-doctor–patient confidentiality is a **legal privilege** granted to patients

-requires physicians to keep patient information private, unless doctor is legally compelled to make disclosure or patient waives privilege

-many gray areas in which a physician's legal and ethical duties may conflict; remote rural settings

-*Jaffee v. Redmond 1996*; U.S. Supreme Court decision recognizing legal privilege b/w patient and psychotherapist

-Health Insurance Portability and Accountability Act (**HIPAA**) of **1996, specific protections for personal health information**

-several **limits on confidentiality**; when patients consent to specific limited disclosures of their information (third-party payment or court proceeding), disclosure may occur

-should be *minimum* information necessary for specific situation, **"need to know"** approach

-patients should be informed of limits to confidentiality when entering tx

-physician may breach patient confidentiality in order to protect third parties in cases of child or elder abuse or threatened violence; *Tarasoff v. Regents of the University of California, 1974 and 1976*

Conservation, Stage of Concrete Operations (7-11 years)

-ability of children to understand concepts of quantity is one of Piaget's most important cognitive developmental theories

-*most* **important sign** that children are *still* in preoperational stage, **NOT** achieved **conservation** or **reversibility**

-*conservation* is ability to recognize that, although the **shape of objects** *may* **change, objects still maintain or conserve other characteristics** that enable them to be **recognized as the same**

-inability to conserve (which is characteristic of preoperational stage) is observed when a child declares that there is more of an object when it changes shape

-*reversibility* is capacity to **understand relation b/w things**; to realize that one thing **can turn into another and back again** (ice and water)

Copropraxia

-sudden, **tic**-like **vulgar, sexual**, or **obscene gesture**

-is a complex motor tic

-clinical evidence suggests that these tics are also observed in neurological disorders that involve **frontostriatal** and **medial prefrontal** lesions

Correctional mental health, "necessaries" doctrine

-fundamental policy is to provide the **same level of mental health services** to each patient in **criminal justice system** that *should* be **available in community system**

-standard is **generally higher** than provided to **law-abiding individuals** *not* incarcerated and is based in *both* **constitutional and common law**

-**"necessaries" doctrine** and subsequent constitutional law make it illegal for jails and prisons to be "deliberately indifferent" to serious medical needs of prisoners

Culturally and Linguistically Appropriate Services (CLAS)

-respond to need to ensure that all **people entering health care system receive equitable** *and* **effective tx** in **culturally and linguistically** *appropriate* manner

-proposed as means to correct inequities that currently exist in the provision of health services and to make these services more responsive to individual needs of all patients/consumers

-standards are **intended to be inclusive of all cultures** *and* **NOT limited to any particular population group** or sets of groups; especially designed to **address needs of racial**, **ethnic**, and **linguistic population groups** that experience *unequal* access to health services

-aim of the standards is to contribute to elimination of racial and ethnic health disparities and to improve health of all Americans

-CLAS standards are primarily directed at health care organizations; however, individual providers are also encouraged to use the standards to make their practices more culturally and linguistically accessible

-there are 14 standards organized by themes: Culturally Competent Care (Standards 1-3), Language Access Services (Standards 4-7), and Organizational Supports for Cultural Competence (Standards 8-14). 3 types of standards of varying stringency: mandates, guidelines, and recommendations

D

Death, Childrens' understanding
-children have a very limited understanding of death

-ideas about death develop along clear developmental lines; grouped by levels of mental functioning

-ideas about death by age group:

6-7 yrs; often magical and eccentric

7-11 yrs; more concrete, may cite causes of death

12 and older, adolescence; capable of more abstract formal reasoning

-many children **< 7 yrs** *may* **fail to recognize** *irreversibility* **of death**

Delirium, pharmacological treatment
-2 major sxs that *may* **require pharmacological tx** are **psychosis** and **insomnia**

-**haloperidol**, a butyrophenone antipsychotic drug is commonly used; depending on age, weight, and physical condition, initial dose may range from 2-6 mg IM, repeated in an hour if patient remains agitated

-2 daily oral doses should suffice, **w/ 2/3 of dose being given at bedtime**; **oral** dose should be ~**1.5 times parenteral dose**

-effective total daily dose of haloperidol may range from 5-40 mg for most patients w/ delirium

-phenothiazines should be avoided in delirious patients because these drugs are a/w significant anticholinergic activity

-**second-generation antipsychotics**, such as risperidone, clozapine, olanzapine, quetiapine, ziprasidone, and aripiprazole, may be considered

-for patients w/ Parkinson's dz and delirium; clozapine or quetiapine have some support in the literature and are less likely to exacerbate parkinsonian sxs

-**insomnia** is best tx'd w/ benzodiazepines w/ short or intermediate half-lives (e.g., lorazepam 1-2 mg at bedtime)

-benzodiazepines w/ long half-lives and barbiturates should be avoided unless being used to tx underlying disorder (e.g., alcohol withdrawal)

-case reports of improvement in or remission of delirious states from intractable medical illnesses w/ **ECT**

Dementia, diagnosis and clinical features

-dx based on clinical examination, including mental status examination, and information from patient's family, friends, and employers

-**memory impairment** is typically an **early and prominent feature** in dementia, especially in **dementias involving the cortex**, such as dementia of **Alzheimer's** type

-**early**, memory impairment is mild; *most* marked for **recent events**

-**later**, memory impairment becomes severe; *only* **earliest learned information is retained**

-no matter how severe disorientation seems, patients show **NO** impairment in **level of consciousness**

-lability of emotions, sloppy grooming, uninhibited remarks, or dull, apathetic, or vacuous facial expression

-dementing processes that affect cortex, primarily dementia of Alzheimer's type and vascular dementia, can affect patients' language abilities

-DSM-IV-TR includes aphasia as criteria; vague, stereotyped, imprecise, or circumstantial locution, as well as difficulty naming objects

Dependent Personality Disorder

-initially described by Abraham (1927) as "oral" character, predecessor of Dependent PD

-thought to result from fixation at the first, or oral, stage of psychosexual development

-personality type was similar to Horney's "compliant" type

-was a subtype of passive-aggressive PD in DSM-I and did not become a separate disorder until DSM-III

-DSM-IV put greater emphasis on the disorder's central features and attempted to diminish its overlap w/ other PDs

-occurs in ~1.25% of general population; much more common among women

-characterized by *excessive* **need to be cared for by others**, which leads to **submissive and clinging behavior** and *excessive* **fears of separation**

-able to care for self but doubt their ability and judgment; **view others as much stronger** and **more capable** than they are

-*excessively* **rely on "powerful" others to initiate and do things for them**, make their decisions, assume responsibility for their actions, and guide them through life

-low self-esteem and doubts about their effectiveness lead them to avoid positions of responsibility

-*may* **go to great lengths to maintain dependent relationships**; may always agree w/ those on whom they depend, and they tend to be excessively passive and self-sacrificing

-**feel incapable of caring for themselves** when relationships end; feel helpless and fearful

-may indiscriminately begin another relationship so that they can be provided w/ direction and nurturance; unfulfilling or even abusive relationship may seem better than being on their own

-dependent persons want others to assume a controlling function that would frighten the borderline patient; individuals w/ DPD become appeasing rather than rageful or self-destructive when threatened w/ separation

-both avoidant and dependent PDs are characterized by low self-esteem, rejection sensitivity, and an excessive need for reassurance; persons w/ DPD seek out rather than avoid relationships, quickly and indiscriminately replace ended relationships

Dialectical Behavior Therapy (DBT), Borderline PD
-type of psychotherapy **originally developed** for *chronically* **self-injurious patients w/borderline PD** and **parasuicidal acts/behavior**

-eclectic, drawing on concepts derived from **supportive**, **cognitive**, and **behavioral** therapies

-some elements can be **traced** to **Franz Alexander's view of therapy as a corrective emotional experience**, and other elements from certain Eastern philosophy

-patients are seen weekly, w/ goal of improving interpersonal skills and decreasing self-destructive behavior using techniques involving advice, metaphor, storytelling, and confrontation, among others

-Marsha **Linehan**, Ph.D., developed the tx method, based on theory that such patients **cannot identify emotional experiences and cannot tolerate frustration or rejection**

-DBT assumes **ALL behavior** (including thoughts and feelings) is **learned**; **behave in ways that reinforce or even reward behavior**, regardless of how maladaptive

-**5 essential "functions" in tx**: (1) enhance and expand patient's repertoire of skillful behavioral patterns; (2) improve patient motivation to change by reducing reinforcement of maladaptive behavior, including dysfunctional cognition and emotion; (3) ensure new behavioral patterns generalize from therapeutic to natural environment; (4) structure environment so that effective behaviors, rather than dysfunctional behaviors, are reinforced; and (5) enhance motivation and capabilities of therapist so that effective tx is rendered

-**4 modes of tx in DBT**: (1) group skills training, (2) individual therapy, (3) phone consultations, and (4) consultation team

-studies w/ borderline PD have been positive; low dropout rate from tx; incidence of **parasuicidal acts/behaviors declined**; self-report of angry affect decreased; and social adjustment and work performance improved

-applied to other disorders, including substance abuse, eating disorders, schizophrenia, and posttraumatic stress disorder

Diphenhydramine, anticholinergic toxicity

-primary side effect of diphenhydramine is sedation; some may cause GI distress

-drying of the mouth and respiratory passages can occur

-**anticholinergic toxicity** is most concerning; **tachycardia** is earliest, most reliable sign, as well as **decreased or absent bowel sounds**

Cutaneous vasodilation; "red as a beet" occurs to compensate for loss of sweat production

Anhidrosis; "dry as a bone" occurs b/c sweat glands are innervated by muscarinic receptors subsequently causing dry skin

Anhydrotic hyperthermia; "hot as a hare" results from interference w/ heat dissipation through sweating leading to hyperthermia

Nonreactive mydriasis; "blind as a bat" results from muscarinic input leading to pupillary dilation and ineffective accommodation; frequently manifests as blurry vision

Delirium; "mad as a hatter" results from blockade of muscarinic receptors in CNS, may include anxiety, agitation, dysarthria, confusion, disorientation, visual hallucinations, bizarre behavior, delirium, psychosis w/paranoia, coma, and seizures; hallucinations often described as people appearing to become larger and smaller, "Lilliputian type" or "Alice in Wonderland-like"

Bladder detrusor muscle and **urethral sphincter conrol**; "full as a flask" results from reduction of detrusor contraction, reducing or eliminating desire to urinate and prevention of normal opening of urethral sphincter leading to urinary retention

Direct conditioning, fear development

-occurs when an individual is frightened by a **single exposure** to **cues a/w intensely aversive event** resulting in person **remaining fearful of those cues**

-described in early conditioning models of fear acquisition; considered part of **environmental learning pathway** of fear development

-**Mowrer's** (1960) **2-factor theory of phobia development** suggests that *excessive* fear is result of a **direct conditioning experience** and its *maintenance* by **avoidant behavior**

-direct conditioning alone does NOT sufficiently explain development of all phobias, including excessive fears

-most effective clinical intervention (exposure therapy) in tx of specific phobias is based on conditioning principles despite controversy surrounding classical conditioning theory for phobias

Discontinuation syndrome, antidepressants

-occurs in ~**20% of patients after abrupt discontinuation** of an antidepressant medication that was taken for **at least 6 wks**

-definitive pathophysiologic explanation remains unknown

-**ALL** approved antidepressants have had case reports or warnings from manufacturers for discontinuation syndrome in response to **abrupt discontinuation or medication tapering**

-typical sxs include **flu-like sxs, insomnia, nausea, imbalance, sensory disturbances,** and **hyperarousal**

-sxs are usually mild, last 1-2 weeks; **rapidly extinguished w/ restarting of antidepressant**

-*more likely* **w/ longer duration of tx** and **shorter half-life** antidepressant

-high index of suspicion should be maintained w/ presence of discontinuation sxs; close questioning should identify accidental or purposeful self-discontinuation of medication

-patient education should include warnings about potential problems a/w abrupt discontinuation

Dissociative Identity Disorder, etiology

-strongly linked to severe, **early childhood trauma** (frequently **physical** and **sexual**)

-rates of reported **severe childhood trauma, 85-97%**

-no current evidence for significant genetic contribution

-disturbed **affect modulation** is common, **mood swings, depression, suicidal** tendency, and generalized **irritability**

-impulse control often impaired, risk-taking, substance abuse, and inappropriate or self-destructive behaviors

-high levels of anxiety and panic are common

-**identity diffusion** seen w/ borderline traits; alter identities reflect disruptions in psychological integration of traumatic and nontraumatic aspects of self

-**eating disorders** are common in subgroup of trauma patients

-frequent **somatization, conversion,** and psychophysiological disorders

-likely to have **lower threshold** for experiencing noxious stimuli or **pain**

Dopamine receptor antagonist overdose

-**thioridazine** and **mesoridazine** have *worst* **prognosis** secondary to **cardiac complications**

-**haloperidol** (w/o ingestion of other substances or alcohol) has ***best*** **prognosis**

-sxs include: EPS, mydriasis, tachycardia, hypotension, decreased DTRs

-*severe* **cases** may include: delirium, respiratory depression, seizure, **coma**

Double Depression and Dysthymic Disorder

-dysthymic disorder (DD); defined as mild, chronic depressive condition, typically characterized by mild-moderate level of depressive sxs

-*almost* **all individuals w/ DD have exacerbations that meet criteria for major depressive episode (MDE), or "double depression"**, at some point (Keller et al., 1995 ; Klein et al., 2006)

-literature on prognostic factors in DD is sparse; generally limited to brief f/u periods

-a 2-year f/u of double depression reported age, marital status, and number and duration of MDEs did NOT predict recovery from DD (Keller et al., 1983)

-a combined retrospective/prospective f/u of depressed children found that **earlier age of onset** (Kovacs et al., 1997) and **comorbid externalizing d/o predicted longer duration of DD**, while sex, superimposed MDE, and comorbid anxiety d/o failed to predict recovery from DD (Kovacs et al., 1997)

-report based on first 5 years of a 10-year naturalistic follow-up study found that **comorbid anxiety d/o, cluster C personality d/o traits, and family hx of bipolar d/o** predicted *lower* **rate of recovery from DD** (Hayden & Klein, 2001)

Double-blind, study design

-helps **eliminate bias** because neither patient nor persons involved in study know which, if any, tx is being given

-in drug studies, a control group of patients may receive a placebo (i.e., inert substance prepared to resemble active drug being tested in experiment)

-response to placebo may represent psychological effect of taking a pill; response is not caused by any psychopharmacological property (placebo effect)

-investigators do not know the tx given because drugs are identified by special codes unknown to them

-outcome may be assessed by persons other than those administering the tx (blind evaluators)

-control subjects may receive an alternative comparison tx, rather than just a placebo

Driving, dementia

-most of available evidence suggests that **dementia, even when mild, impairs driving performance** to some extent

-**risk of accidents *increases* w/ increasing severity of dementia**

-studies demonstrate more difficulties comprehending and operating driving simulator, drove off the road more often, spent more time driving considerably slower than posted speed limit, applied less brake pressure in stop zones, spent more time negotiating left turns, and drove more poorly overall

-impossible to assess in office or hospital setting; neuropsychiatric impairments or behavioral sxs on driving performance is neither clear-cut nor predictive

-risks of driving should be discussed w/ all patients w/ dementia and their families, and these **discussions should be carefully documented**

-should include exploration of patient's current driving patterns, transportation needs, and potential alternatives; should ask family about any hx of getting lost, traffic accidents, or near accidents

-issue should be raised repeatedly and reassessed over time

-no clear consensus regarding threshold level of dementia at which driving should be curtailed or discontinued

-evidence-based review of driving and Alzheimer's dz from American Academy of Neurology found that driving was only mildly impaired in drivers w/ Clinical Dementia Rating (CDR) of 0.5 (mild cognitive impairment), but those w/ CDR of 1 (mild or early stage dementia) were found to pose significant risks from increased vehicular accidents and poorer driving

-additional increases in risk may also be a/w dx of dementia w/ Lewy bodies

-w/ moderate impairment (e.g., those who cannot perform moderately complex tasks, such as preparing simple meals, household chores, yard work, or simple home repairs), there is some evidence and strong clinical consensus that driving poses an unacceptable risk and patients should be instructed not to drive

-w/ severe impairment; generally unable to drive and certainly should not do so

-psychiatrists ***should* familiarize themselves w/ state motor vehicle regulations** for **reporting individuals w/ dementia**

-disclosure is **forbidden in some states; other states require reporting** of the dx of dementia or Alzheimer's dz to the state department of motor vehicles; **patient and family *should* be informed**

-in many states, the physician may breach confidentiality to inform the state motor vehicle department of a patient who is judged to be a dangerous driver

Drug interactions

-occurs when **pharmacological action of a medication is altered by concurrently administered drug** (or exogenous substance)

-**3 main types** of drug interactions are *pharmacokinetic* **interactions**, *pharmacodynamic* **interactions**, and *idiosyncratic* **interactions**

-**pharmacodynamic** interactions occur when **action of a drug changes at a receptor or biologically active site**, which **alters pharmacological effect** of a given plasma concentration of the drug

-**pharmacokinetic** interactions occur when **one medication alters pharmacokinetics** (absorption, distribution, metabolism, or excretion) of another drug

-**idiosyncratic** interactions **occur unpredictably in a small number of patients**; are unexpected, given known pharmacological actions of individual drugs

E

Emergent suicidality risk factors

-acute risk factors are much more predictive than chronic risk factors

-include *increasing* **anxiety** and **frank panic attacks, psychic turmoil, global insomnia**, mood-congruent **nihilistic delusions**, *profound* **hopelessness**, and *recent* **discharge** from **psychiatric hospital** (Busch et al. 2003; Fawcett 1992; Fawcett et al. 1991)

-individuals experiencing the first 3 of these sxs should be viewed as being particularly high risk regardless of whether they verbalize suicidal ideation

-the 3-month period following discharge poses a significant period of vulnerability; one population study demonstrated 7.8% of suicide victims completed suicide w/in 1 month of discharge (Deisenhammer et al. 2007)

Encopresis, treatment

-according to DSM-IV-TR, repeated passage of feces into inappropriate places (e.g., clothing or floor) whether involuntary or intentional; **at least one such event a month** for **at least 3 months**; chronological age is **at least 4 years** (or *equivalent* developmental level); behavior is not due exclusively to direct physiological effects of substance (e.g., laxatives) or a general medical condition except through a mechanism involving constipation

-despite frequency of childhood encopresis, **no large, RCTs** have been conducted

-tx remains **largely experiential** than evidence based

-generally consists of **psychoeducation**; colonic evacuation followed by routine **laxative** tx; and **toilet training** which is composed of regularly scheduled toileting, maintenance of symptom diary, and age-appropriate incentive scheme

-aim of approach is to decrease physical and emotional distress a/w defecation; develop or restore normal bowel habits w/ positive reinforcement; and encourage child and parents to take active role during tx

Erikson's Stages of Psychosocial Development, related psychopathology

-represent **continuum** of development

-**internal crises** *triggered* by combination of physical, cognitive, instinctual, and sexual changes; **resolution** results in **growth and development** *or* **psychosocial regression**

Stage 1, **Trust vs. Mistrust** (Birth-18 mos)

-psychosis, addictions, depression

Stage 2, **Autonomy vs. Shame and Doubt** (~18 mos-~3 yrs)

-paranoia, obsessions, compulsions, impulsivity

Stage 3, **Initiative vs. Guilt** (~3 yrs-~5 yrs)

-conversion d/o, phobia, psychosomatic d/o, inhibition

Stage 4, **Industry vs. Inferiority** (~5 yrs-~13 yrs)

-creative inhibition, inertia

Stage 5, **Identity vs. Role Confusion** (~13 yrs-~21 yrs)

-delinquent behavior, gender-related identity d/o, borderline psychotic episodes

Stage 6, **Intimacy vs. Isolation** (~21 yrs-~40 yrs)

-schizoid personality d/o, distantiation

Stage 7, **Generativity vs. Stagnation** (~40 yrs-~60 yrs)

-mid-life crisis, premature invalidism

Stage 8, **Integrity vs. Despair** (~60 yrs-Death)

-extreme alienation, despair

F

Facilitation

-interview technique that uses **encouraging comments** to draw attention to patient's feelings; **helps patient focus** while **relating events and feelings** during an interview or psychotherapy

Female Hypoactive Sexual Desire Disorder, biological treatments

-**hormonal** therapy; based on androgen levels in women declining after menopause, frequently report low sexual desire; **not FDA**-approved

-low doses of testosterone have been studied to improve sexual functioning, increasing libido and sense of well-being; pose some risks including hirsutism, deepening of the voice, acne, and enlargement of clitoris; positive association b/w androgen levels and breast cancer has been reported

-**nonhormonal** therapy; phosphodiesterase-5 inhibitors (sildenafil, tadalafil, vardenafil), no solid evidence

-**bupropion** hydrochloride; **limited evidence** from 2 small studies that antidepressant w/ dopaminergic and adrenergic properties might be useful in nondepressed women w/ Female Hypoactive Sexual Desire Disorder

Femoral nerve lesion
Sensory supply

-antero-medial surface of thigh and leg to medial malleolus

Sensory loss

-usually corresponds to distribution

Area of pain

-anterior thigh and medial leg

Reflex arc

-knee jerk

Motor deficit

-extension of knee

Source of lesion

-DM, femoral hernia, femoral artery aneurysm, posterior abdominal neoplasm, psoas abscess, trauma

Festinating gait

-gait disturbance characterized by **involuntarily acceleration**

-movement w/ **short**, **jerky**, **steps** and often on **tiptoe**

-suspect **Parkinson's** if it accompanies **postural instability** and **truncal rigidity**

Fetal Alcohol Syndrome

-occurs **~1 in 3,000 live births**

-prevalence in **alcoholic mothers, 2.5-10%**

In utero alcohol exposure and:

1. **intrauterine growth retardation**

2. **microcephaly**, **microphthalmia**, **short palpebral fissures**, **midface hypoplasia**, **thin upper lip**, **long philtrum**

3. delayed development, hyperactivity, attention deficits, intellectual delays, learning disabilities, occasional seizures

4. persistent postnatal poor growth in weight and height

-children born to alcoholic mothers w/o FAS demonstrate intellectual impairment, decreased birth weight, congenital anomalies

-**leading nongenetic cause** of **mental retardation** in U.S.

Fiduciary; doctor-patient relationship

-person **who acts for another** in a capacity that involves a **confidence or trust**

-derives from the Latin word for "confidence" or "trust"

Fixed-ratio schedule

-**reinforcement** schedule in which a reward is given after a **specific number responses** have been emitted

Flooding

-sometimes called *implosion*; works **best w/ specific phobias**

-similar to graded exposure; involves **exposing patient to feared object** *in vivo*; no hierarchy

-based on premise that **escaping from anxiety-provoking experience** *reinforces* **anxiety through conditioning**

-can **extinguish anxiety** and **prevent conditioned avoidance** behavior by **not allowing** patients to *escape the situation*

-encourage patients to confront feared situations directly, w/o gradual buildup, as in systematic desensitization or graded exposure

-no relaxation exercises are used, as in systematic desensitization

-patients experience fear, which gradually subsides after a time

-success of procedure depends on having patients remain in fear-generating situation until they are calm and feel a sense of mastery

-prematurely withdrawing from situation or prematurely terminating fantasized scene is equivalent to an escape, which then reinforces both the conditioned anxiety and the avoidance behavior; produces the opposite of the desired effect

-in a variant, called *imaginal flooding*, feared object or situation is **confronted only in imagination**, not in real life

-many patients refuse flooding because of psychological discomfort involved

-it is also contraindicated when intense anxiety would be hazardous to patient (heart dz or fragile psychological adaptation)

Fluoxetine, children and adolescents

-**approved** for **tx of depression** in children **8-17 yrs** and **OCD** in children **ages 7-17 yrs**

-**meta-analysis of published and unpublished studies** on use of SSRIs for pediatric depression concluded *only* fluoxetine had *favorable* **risk-benefit profile**

-except for fluoxetine, risks of tx w/ SSRIs considered greater than potential benefits

G

Gender Identity Disorder, diagnosis
-first introduced in DSM-III

-term *transsexualism* was eliminated in DSM-IV

-2 necessary components of gender identity disorder:

strong and *persistent* **cross-gender identification** (NOT merely a desire for any perceived cultural advantages of being the other sex)

persistent *discomfort* **w/ one's sex** or **sense of** *inappropriateness* **in gender role** of that sex

-dx is NOT given if person has concurrent physical condition, partial androgen insensitivity syndrome or congenital adrenal hyperplasia

-MUST be evidence of clinically significant distress or impairment

Generalized Anxiety Disorder, diagnostic features
-**anxiety** and **worry** in excess about a number of events, apprehensive expectation

-**no** (difficulty) **controlling worry**

-duration; **more days than not** for **at least 6 months**

-anxiety and worry are accompanied by **at least 3 additional sxs**:

Irritability

Concentrating, difficulty

Restlessness

Energy (easily fatigued)

Sleep, disturbed

Tension, muscle

-*only* **1 additional symptom** is required in **children**

-focus of the anxiety and worry is not confined to features of another Axis I d/o

-individuals report subjective distress d/t constant worry; difficulty controlling worry; or impairment in social, occupational, or important areas of functioning

-not d/t direct physiological effects of substance or a general medical condition and does not occur exclusively during a Mood D/O, Psychotic D/O, or Pervasive Developmental D/O

-intensity, duration, or frequency of anxiety and worry is far out of proportion to actual likelihood or impact of feared event

-person finds it difficult to keep worrisome thoughts from interfering w/ attention to tasks at hand and has difficulty stopping the worry

-adults often worry about every day, routine life circumstances such as possible job responsibilities, finances, health of family members, misfortune to their children, or minor matters

-children tend to worry excessively about competence or quality of performance

-during course of disorder, focus of worry may shift from one concern to another

Genetic anticipation
-phenomenon in which a **genetic dz appears** *earlier* and w/ *greater* severity in each **successive generation** in a pedigree

-seen in **Huntington dz, myotonic dystrophy**; also occurs in **fragile X** syndrome

-d/t **expansion** of **trinucleotide repeat** sequence in DNA

Grounds for Termination of Parental Rights
-specific circumstances under which the **child cannot safely be returned home** because of **risk of harm by the parent** or **inability** of the parent to provide for the child's basic needs

-each State is responsible for establishing its own statutory grounds; these **vary by State**

-**most common** statutory grounds for determining **parental *unfitness*** include:

Severe or chronic **abuse** *or* **neglect**

Abuse or neglect of ***other* children** in the household

Abandonment

Long-term mental illness or deficiency of the parent(s)

Long-term alcohol- or drug-induced incapacity of the parent(s)

Failure to support or maintain contact w/ the child

Involuntary termination of the rights of the parent to *another* child

-another common ground for termination is a **felony conviction** of the parent(s) for a crime of violence against the child or another family member, or a conviction for any felony when the term of incarceration is so long as to have a negative impact on the child, and the only available provision of care for the child is foster care

H

Hallucinogen intoxication

-interferes w/ **serotonin** neurotransporters

-induces **euphoria** in addition to **delusions** and **visual hallucinations**

-**perceptual changes** are the hallmark of use and occur in state of **full wakefulness and alertness**; include depersonalization, derealization, illusions, hallucinations, synesthesias

-psychological effects can be unpredictable; may be influenced by user's mindset prior to intoxication and setting of use

-can be marked by feelings of intense fear w/ avoidant responses

-physical effects include increased body temperature, pupillary dilation, tachycardia, sweating, palpitations, vision blurring, tremors, incoordination

Haloperidol, chorea and abnormal involuntary movements a/w Huntington dz

-"chorea" is a borrowed Latin word that derives from Greek khoreia, a choral dance; basic Greek word for dance (written w/ Roman alphabet) is khoros

-Committee on Classification of the World Federation of Neurology has defined chorea as "a state of **excessive**, **spontaneous movements**, **irregularly timed**, **non-repetitive**, **randomly distributed** and **abrupt in character**. These movements may vary in severity from restlessness w/ mild intermittent exaggeration of gesture and expression, fidgeting movements of the hands, unstable dance-like gait to a continuous flow of disabling, violent movements"

-exhibit motor impersistence (ie, **cannot maintain a sustained posture**); when attempting to grip an object, they **alternately squeeze and release** ('milkmaid's grip'); when they attempt to protrude the **tongue**, it *often* **pops in and out** ('harlequin's tongue')

-*often* **drop objects involuntarily**; common are attempts by patients to mask chorea by voluntarily augmenting the choreiform movements w/ semipurposeful movements

-involves *both* **proximal and distal muscles**; normal tone is noted, but, in some instances, hypotonia is present; in movement d/o centers, **levodopa**-*induced* chorea is **most common movement d/o**, followed by Huntington dz

-Huntington chorea, content of **striatal dopamine is normal**, indicating that major pathological alterations lay in surviving, but diseased, medium-sized, spiny, striatal dopaminergic neurons

-pharmacologic agents that *either* **deplete dopamine** (eg, reserpine and tetrabenazine) or **block dopamine receptors** (eg, neuroleptic medications) *improve* chorea

-increasing amount of dopamine worsens chorea, such as in levodopa-induced chorea seen w/ Parkinson dz

-only symptomatic tx is available for patients w/ chorea

-most widely used agents in tx of chorea are neuroleptics; **haloperidol**, fluphenazine, atypical

Hemiballismus

-**intermittent flinging of arm and leg**, gross movements of one side of the body

-movements are violent, less predictable, unilateral, and consist of flinging of proximal body parts

-originally, **a/w lesions** in *contralateral* **subthalamic nucleus**

-**recent** studies, thought to be lesions in **caudate nucleus** or other **basal ganglia**

-**NO cognitive impairment**, **paresis**, or **corticospinal tract signs**

-**most common** etiology in individuals **> 65 yo**, occlusion of small perforating branch of basilar artery causing **stroke in basal ganglia**

-in HIV, toxoplasmosis lesions tend to develop in basal ganglia

-lesion also seen w/ vasculitis

-few treatments; dopamine-blocking antipsychotics can suppress movements

Herpes simplex encephalitis, clinical features

-**most frequent** cause of **serious, nonepidemic** encephalitis

-predilection for **frontal inferior surface** of the brain and attacks **undersurface of both frontal and temporal lobes**

-causes **fever, somnolence,** and **delirium** (hallucinations)

-causes **partial complex seizures** and **memory impairment** (temporal lobe and limbic system)

-causes **language** *impairment* and **behavior** *changes*, including **irritability** (frontal lobes)

-human variant Klüver-Bucy syndrome has been described w/ bilateral temporal lobe involvement

Histrionic Personality Disorder, neurotic vs. primitive

Neurotic (hysterical) variant

-**Restrained** and circumscribed emotionality

-Sexualized exhibitionism and *need to be loved*

-*Good* impulse control

-**Subtly appealing** seductiveness

-Ambition and competitiveness

-**Mature,** triangular object relations

-Separations from love objects *can be tolerated*

-Strict superego and some obsessional defenses

-Sexualized transference wishes *develop gradually* and are viewed as *unrealistic*

Primitive variant

-**Florid** and generalized emotionality

-Greedy exhibitionism w/ *demanding* quality that is "cold" and less engaging

-*May* become **impulsive** under stress

-**Crude**, **inappropriate**, and **distancing** seductiveness

-Aimlessness and helplessness

-**Primitive**, dyadic object relations characterized by clinging, masochism, and paranoia

-*Overwhelming* **separation anxiety** when *abandoned* by love objects

-Lax superego w/ proneness to rely on primitive defenses, such as **splitting** and **idealization**, when under stress

-Intense sexualized transference wishes *develop rapidly* and are viewed as *realistic* expectations

HIV-Related Dementia

-encephalopathy in HIV infection is a/w dementia, termed AIDS dementia complex, or HIV dementia

-patients infected w/ HIV experience dementia at **annual rate of ~14%**

- **~75%** of patients w/ AIDS have **CNS involvement** at the time of **autopsy**

-development of **dementia** is *often* **paralleled by appearance of parenchymal abnormalities** on MRI

-other infectious dementias, caused by Cryptococcus or Treponema pallidum

-dx made by **confirmation of HIV infection** and **exclusion of alternative pathology**

-cognitive, motor, and behavioral changes are assessed using physical, neurological, and psychiatric examinations, in addition to neuropsychological testing

-AIDS Task Force criteria for AIDS dementia complex:

Laboratory evidence for systemic HIV

At least **2 cognitive deficits**

Presence of **motor abnormalities** or **personality changes**; may be apathy, emotional lability, or behavioral disinhibition

Absence **of clouding of consciousness** or **evidence of *another* etiology** that could produce cognitive impairment

Huntington's Disease, clinical features

-**incurable**, **adult-onset**, **autosomal dominant** inherited disorder a/w cell loss w/in specific subset of neurons in basal ganglia and cortex

-neuropathology occurs w/in **neostriatum**, gross atrophy of caudate nucleus and putamen accompanied by selective neuronal loss and astrogliosis

-marked neuronal loss also seen in deep layers of cerebral cortex; globus pallidus, thalamus, subthalamic nucleus, substantia nigra, cerebellum show varying degrees of atrophy

-clinical features include **movement disorder**, **cognitive d/o**, and **behavioral d/o**

-**chorea** is characteristic feature, initially may pass for fidgetiness

-**bradykinesia** and akinesia are frequent features

-**dystonia**, sustained muscle contractions

-**eye movement abnormalities** can be seen *early*

-**tendon reflexes** are variable, reduced to pathologically brisk w/ clonus

-**hyperkinesias**, tics and myoclonus may be seen

-**dementia**; early onset **behavioral changes**, irritability, untidiness, loss of interest

-**depression**, increased rate of suicide; can develop psychosis, obsessive-compulsive sxs, sexual and sleep disturbances, changes in personality

Hydrocephalus, symptoms

-disturbance of **formation**, **flow**, or **absorption** of cerebrospinal fluid (CSF) that leads to an increase in volume occupied by CSF in CNS

-**acute** hydrocephalus occurs **over days**; **subacute** hydrocephalus occurs **over weeks**; and **chronic** hydrocephalus occurs **over months or years**

-cerebral atrophy and focal destructive lesions also lead to abnormal increase of CSF in CNS; loss of cerebral tissue leaves vacant space that is filled passively w/CSF and are NOT classified as hydrocephalus (formerly described as hydrocephalus ex vacuo)

-Symptoms in adults

Cognitive *deterioration*

Headaches; more prominent in AM because CSF is resorbed less efficiently in recumbent position; rarely present in NPH

Neck pain; if present, may indicate protrusion of cerebellar tonsils into foramen magnum

Nausea; not exacerbated by head movements

Vomiting; sometimes explosive, is more significant in AM

Blurred vision (and episodes of 'graying out'); may suggest serious optic nerve compromise; should be treated as emergency

Double vision (horizontal diplopia); **sixth nerve palsy**

Difficulty in **walking**

Drowsiness

Incontinence (**urinary** *first*, fecal later if untreated); indicates significant destruction of frontal lobes and advanced dz

Hypochondriasis, clinical description

-characterized by **6 months or more** of general and nondelusional **preoccupation w/ fears** of having, or **idea** that one has, a **serious dz** based on person's **misinterpretation of bodily sxs**

-preoccupation causes significant distress and impairment in one's life; it is not accounted for by another psychiatric or medical disorder

-essential feature in hypochondriasis is preoccupation **NOT w/ sxs themselves** but rather w/ the **fear or idea of having a serious dz**

-preoccupation persists despite evidence to the contrary and reassurance from physicians

-subset of individuals w/ hypochondriasis has poor insight about presence of this disorder

-term hypochondriasis is derived from the old medical term hypochondrium, "below the ribs;" reflects common abdominal complaints of many patients w/ the disorder although sxs may occur in any part of body

I

Impaired physician, substance use disorder

- ~**10-15%** of all healthcare professionals will **misuse drugs or alcohol** at some time during their career

-rates of substance abuse and dependence are similar to those of general population

-*higher* **rates of abuse** w/ **benzodiazepines** and **opiates**

-**anesthesia, emergency medicine**, and **psychiatry** have higher rates of substance abuse

-**alcohol** is **most commonly misused**, followed by **opioids** and **stimulants**, such as cocaine

-risk for **men** developing substance abuse is significantly higher than for women in both the overall population and in healthcare professionals

Infant temperament, anxiety disorder

-Kagan et al. studied **temperamental** category termed **"reactivity"**

-observed physiologic and behavioral traits linked to variations in amygdalar responses

-**behaviorally inhibited** children appear to have **over-reactive amygdala**, triggering highly responsive sympathetic nervous system when confronted w/ stressful stimuli

-4 month-old infants who became "motorically aroused" and distressed to novel stimuli were termed highly reactive; infants that remained "motorically relaxed" and did not cry were termed low reactive

-infants were tested again at 14 and 21 months; **highly reactive** infants were characterized by high fear to unfamiliar events, termed *inhibited*

-low reactive children were minimally fearful to novel situations, characterized by as uninhibited

-at age 4 ½, most children did not maintain their expected profile d/t subsequent experiences and family interventions

-children that **remained highly inhibited** or uninhibited after 4 ½ yrs were at *higher* risk for developing **anxiety** and conduct d/o, respectively

Informed Consent, 3 Requirements

1. **Competency** (intelligence)

-Incompetence refers to a court adjudication, whereas incapacity indicates a functional inability as determined by a clinician

-standard for determining competence includes: Communication of choice; Understanding of relevant information provided; Appreciation of available options and consequences; Rational decision making

2. **Information** (knowing)

-"material" information that a reasonable person in patient's position would want to know to make informed decision; *Canterbury v. Spence, 1972*

3. **Voluntariness**

-must be given freely by the patient and w/o coercion, fraud, or duress

-**2 basic exceptions** informed consent:

1. immediate tx is necessary to **save a life or prevent serious harm**, and it is not possible to obtain either patient's consent or that of someone authorized to provide consent for patient

2. therapeutic privilege, excepts informed consent if a psychiatrist determines that **complete disclosure of possible risks and alternatives** *might* have **deleterious impact on patient's health and welfare**; jurisdictions vary in application of this exception

Interferon, side effects and neuropsychiatric symptoms

-substantial side effects complicate tx

-majority of patients receiving interferon-based therapy experience side effects, including fatigue, muscle aches, influenza-like sxs, GI disturbances, hematologic abnormalities, and neuropsychiatric sxs

-side effects are generally proportionate to tx dose and duration; noted w/ all types of interferon tx

-intolerability caused by neuropsychiatric side effects leads to discontinuation of interferon in up to 13% of cases

-**most common neuropsychiatric side effects** are **fatigue** and **depressive sxs**, although a variety of other clinical sxs have been noted

- ~20-40% of chronic hepatitis C patients tx'd w/ interferon suffer from sxs of depression, often necessitating discontinuation of tx

-**suicidal thoughts and actions** have also been reported

-other neuropsychiatric side effects include **panic and anxiety**, **emotional lability**, **irritability**, **anger**, **aggression**, **hypomania and mania**, and **confusion and disorientation**

-rare, psychosis (w/ hallucinations and delusions) is a possible complication of interferon-based tx regimens for hepatitis C

Intermittent Explosive Disorder, etiology

-correlated to **low brain serotonin turnover rate**, **low** concentration of 5-hydroxyindoleacetic acid (**5-HIAA**) **in CSF**; SSRIs and TCAs appear to alleviate sxs

-5-HIAA appears to act on suprachiasmatic nucleus in hypothalamus, target for serotonergic output from dorsal and median raphe nuclei

-low 5-HIAA may be hereditary

-low vagal tone and increased insulin secretion traits correlate w/ IED

-polymorphism of gene for tryptophan hydroxylase, serotonin precursor, has been suggested; genotype is more common w/ impulsive behavior

-may be a/w lesions in prefrontal cortex and amygdale

Interpersonal psychotherapy, Major Depressive Disorder and Social Phobia

-**time-limited** tx developed in 1970s for adult outpatients w/ major depression by Gerald L. **Klerman**, M.D., and Myrna M. **Weissman**, Ph.D.

-straightforward, **manual-based**, focused, pragmatic, and optimistic time-limited tx that **targets particular psychiatric disorders**

-first devised and best tested as tx of **MDE**

-2 basic premises:

1) **depression is a medical illness** that is treatable and not patient's fault

2) disorder does not occur in a vacuum but rather is **influenced by and itself affects the patient's psychosocial environment**

-goal of tx is to help patient **solve difficulty** in his or her **role functioning or social environment**

1) Relieves **sxs**

2) Improves the patient's **environment**

3) Builds **social skills**

4) Fosters a **sense of mastery over the environment**

Interpersonal theory, Harry Stack Sullivan

-Sullivan proposed that patients could keep certain *aspects* or *components* of their **interpersonal relationships out of their awareness** by psychological behavior described as *selective inattention*

-emphasized that analyses should **focus on patients' relationships and personal interactions** to obtain knowledge of affecting patterns and tendencies

-such analyses would consist of detailed questioning regarding moment-to-moment personal interactions, even including those w/ the analyst himself

Involuntary Hospitalization

-limited to **statutorily defined criteria** in all states

-based on the state's decision to exercise its constitutional authority, all states have authorized civil commitment of **individuals who are mentally ill** and **dangerous to self or others**, and *some* states also permit commitment of individuals who are **mentally ill *and* unable to provide for their basic needs**

-each state spells out which criteria are required and what each means

-terms such as *mentally ill* are often loosely described, thus placing responsibility for appropriate dx on clinical judgment of the petitioner

-*some* states have enacted legislation that permits involuntary hospitalization of **3 *other* distinct groups** in addition to individuals w/ mental illness: **developmentally disabled**, **substance-addicted**, and **mentally disabled minors**

-special commitment provisions may exist governing requirements for admission and discharge of mentally disabled minors as well as numerous due-process rights afforded these individuals (*Parham v. J.R. 1979*)

-involuntary hospitalization of psychiatric patients usually arises when **violent behavior threatens to erupt toward self or others** and when patients become **unable to care for themselves**

-frequently manifest mental disorders and conditions that meet substantive criteria for involuntary hospitalization

-**courts, NOT clinicians**, have the **authority to commit patients**

-psychiatrist initiates process that brings patient before the court, usually after a brief period of hospitalization for evaluation or after an evaluation of a prospective patient at request of the court

-psychiatrist must be guided by the tx needs of the patient in seeking involuntary hospitalization, w/in the constraints of commitment standards

-commitment statutes do NOT require involuntary hospitalization but are permissive (Appelbaum et al. 1989); statutes enable MH professionals and others to seek involuntary hospitalization for persons who meet certain substantive criteria

-**duty to seek involuntary hospitalization** is a **standard-of-care issue**; patients who are mentally ill and pose a serious threat to themselves or others may require involuntary hospitalization as a **primary psychiatric intervention**

Isolation of affect

-characteristic of the orderly, controlled persons, often labeled **obsessive-compulsive personalities**

-unlike histrionic personality, individuals w/ obsessive-compulsive personality **remember the truth in fine detail but w/o affect**

-*in crisis*, patients *may* show **intensified self-restraint, overly formal social behavior**, and **obstinacy**

-quests for control may annoy clinicians or make them anxious

-respond well to precise, systematic, and rational explanations

-value efficiency, cleanliness, and punctuality as much as clinicians' effective responsiveness

-should allow such patients to *control* their own care and should **not** engage in a *battle of wills*

K

Kohut's Self psychology, empathic validation

-**empathic validation** is frequently a/w **self psychology**; cornerstone of technique

-all theoretical models of dynamic psychotherapy require some degree of empathic validation to make the patient feel understood and helped

-cognitive and dialectical behavioral therapies have specifically incorporated validating and explaining to patients the childhood origins of their disordered personality functioning

-validation is essential for some narcissistic patients; need to be taught that evolution of character traits is inevitable consequence of development

-narcissistic patients often are unaware of or deny problematic or painful experiences during childhood; may be able to identify negative aspects of their parents' tx

-patients must be persuaded that, considering their development difficulties, their personality styles are really very good, even superior to what might have been alternatives—psychosis or addiction, for instance

-validation also serves to reduce feelings of shame, self-criticism, and self-blame

Kuebler-Ross Model

-originally introduced by Elisabeth Kuebler-Ross (1969)

-also known as **5 stages of grief** are as follows:

1. **Denial**

2. **Anger**

3. **Bargaining**

4. **Depression**

5. **Acceptance**

-*originally* applied to individuals suffering from a **terminal illness**

-do not necessarily occur in order, nor do all stages occur in every patient

Lewy Body Disease; risperidone sensitivity

-second only to Alzheimer's dz as a cause of dementia (McKeith et al. 2004)

-a progressive and often rapidly disabling dementia w/ early (differentiates from Parkinson's) and prominent attentional impairment, executive dysfunction, and visuospatial difficulties

-3 core clinical features:

motor features of Parkinson's dz; *fluctuating* **cognitive function**;

persistent **well-formed visual hallucinations** (often people or animals)

-myoclonus, *absence* of **resting tremor**, and *lack of response* to **L-dopa** are as much as 10x more common in DLB than Parkinson's dz (Louis et al. 1997)

-response to dopaminergic therapies is generally less robust in DLB than in Parkinson's dz (Louis et al. 1997)

-evidence supports use of all presently available acetylcholinesterase (AChE) inhibitors for tx of cognitive impairments in DLB (Edwards et al. 2004)

-AChE inhibitors may improve cognitive features of DLB and hallucinations, delusions, and other neurobehavioral disturbances produced by this condition

-visual hallucinations may predict cognitive response to tx w/ rivastigmine (McKeith et al. 2004)

-some patients may also require tx w/ antipsychotic agents

-particularly susceptible to the adverse effects of typical antipsychotics, including neuroleptic malignant syndrome

-susceptibility may also extend to tx w/ atypical antipsychotic **risperidone** (McKeith et al. 1995)

-quetiapine, **olanzapine**, and **clozapine** are *preferred*

Lithium and ECT, pronlonged seizure and confusion

-may result in **prolonged confusion**, **disorientation**, **speech difficulty**, and **seizures following ECT**

-when brain experiences a seizure (spontaneous or electrically induced), there is massive, widespread depolarization that is characterized by opening of the sodium spike channel

-if Li should be present in the extracellular fluid (patient on maintenance lithium), Li entry would be facilitated

-if the seizure is prolonged or recurrent, toxic intracellular levels may result

-serum Li levels would not rise and may even fall

-cerebellum and spinal cord are affected only secondarily by the seizure, no significant influx of Li would occur, and ataxia or spasticity would be absent

-additionally, if neuromuscular blockers prevent neuromuscular system from participating in the seizure, tremors and fasciculations would not be seen

-signs of Li toxicity would be limited to the cerebrum and would be manifest by altered mental status, disorientation, confusion, speech difficulties (receptive, expressive, or both), and seizures

-discontinuation of Li would be expected to result in improvement over one to several days

-reinstitution of either Li or ECT alone would not result in any deleterious side effects

Lithium levels

-**therapeutic level** in tx of acute mania, **0.8 to 1.5 mEq/L**

-**maintenance level** after acute mania episode, **0.6 to 0.9 mEq/L**

-stable, **steady state levels** are obtained *after* **4-5 days** of initiating or adjusting dose

-levels are generally drawn **12 hrs after last dose**

-levels should be drawn **every 1-3 months during maintenance** therapy

-levels are **altered** dramatically in **pregnancy**, **post-partum**, w/ use of **thiazide diuretic**, **dehydration**, or worsening **renal function**

Lithium toxicity, management

-should immediately contact personal physician; go to hospital ED

-lithium should be **discontinued**; patient should **ingest fluids** if possible

-physical examination (including checking of vital signs) and neuro exam (complete formal MSE) should be performed

-**lithium** and **serum electrolyte levels** should be measured, **renal function tests** performed, and **ECG** obtained

-residual gastric contents should be removed by induction of **emesis**, **gastric lavage**, and absorption w/ **activated charcoal**

-vigorous hydration and maintenance of electrolyte balance are essential

-w/ serum lithium level **> 4.0 mEq/L** or w/ serious manifestations of lithium toxicity, **hemodialysis** should be initiated

-repeat dialysis may be required **every 6-10 hrs, until lithium level is w/in nontoxic range** and **no signs or sxs of lithium toxicity**

Lithium, drug interaction toxicity

-any medication that **alters renal function** can affect lithium levels

-**thiazide diuretics** and **NSAIDs** may *increase* lithium levels by *decreasing* **renal clearance of lithium**

-**angiotensin-converting enzyme inhibitors** and **cyclooxygenase-2 inhibitors** may *increase* **lithium levels**

-drugs that may *decrease* lithium levels include **theophylline** and **aminophylline**

-lithium may potentiate effects of succinylcholine-like muscle relaxants

Lithium, psoriasis exacerbation

-reported prevalence of cutaneous side effects w/ lithium varies from 3.4-45%

-**psoriasis and psoriasiform rash** are among major cutaneous side effects of Li and have resulted in severe emotional distress and noncompliance in bipolar patients tx'd w/ Li

-mechanism by which Li induces or exacerbates psoriasis is not exactly known; role in modulating second messenger systems, adenyl cyclase and inositol monophosphatase–mediated pathways, resulting in alteration in calcium homeostasis; its effect on serotonergic function have been implicated

-NOT all patients w/ preexisting psoriasis will develop a flare in lesions on Li tx

-**psoriasis is NOT considered a contraindication** to Li therapy in bipolar patients

-first description of Li tx a/w psoriasis was by Carter in 1972; several reports of Li-induced psoriasis or exacerbation of preexisting psoriasis have been published

-Li-provoked psoriasis was first reported in 1976 by Bakker and Pepplinkhuizen

-**incidence of psoriasis secondary to Li tx** has been reported to be **1.8-6%**

-common presentation of psoriasis secondary to Li tx is typical plaque-type lesions; other manifestations include pustular psoriasis; fingernail abnormalities; erythroderma; nonspecific psoriasiform dermatitis; and psoriatic arthropathy

-psoriasis induced or exacerbated by Li could be managed w/ conventional tx methods such as topical steroids, keratolytics, vitamin D analogues, oral retinoids, PUVA (psoralen and ultraviolet A) therapy, and methotrexate; **most often these txs may not be very effective**

-**inositol supplementation** was found to be beneficial for psoriasis in patients taking Li compared to those not taking Li in a randomized, double-blind, placebo-controlled crossover trial; related to lithium's "inositol depletion hypothesis" in pathogenesis of Li-induced psoriasis

Lithium, anti-suicidal effects

-**several meta-analyses** have shown **anti-suicidal effects of lithium** and in patients w/ mood disorders

-Cipriani et al. reviewed randomized controlled trials that primarily compared lithium w/ placebo in long-term prophylactic tx for mood disorders; patients who received lithium were less likely to die by suicide (odds ratio = 0.26; 95% confidence interval = 0.09-0.77)

-in reported studies, serum lithium was maintained at so-called therapeutic levels (0.4-1.2 mmol/L)

Lorazepam, absorption PO & IM

-*only* benzodiazepine that is **reliably absorbed** when administered IM

-remains rational choice when treating **acute episode of agitation**; especially when etiology is not clear (hx of schizophrenia *but* may be withdrawing from EtOH)

-**half-life is short** (10-20 hrs) and its route of elimination produces no active metabolites

-usual dosage of 0.5-2.0 mg every 1-6 hrs may be administered PO, SL, IM, or IV

-**respiratory depression** may be a complication in vulnerable patients (obese smokers w/ pulmonary dz)

-**NOT recommended for long-term daily use** because of problems a/w tolerance, dependence, and withdrawal

-concern over **paradoxic** reactions to benzodiazepines; hostility or violence may be exaggerated

Lysergic acid diethylamide (LSD) and other hallucinogens, receptor agonism

-most hallucinogenic substances vary in pharmacological effects

-pharmacodynamic effect of LSD remains controversial although generally agreed that it acts on **serotonergic** system, either as an antagonist or agonist

-current studies suggest, LSD and other hallucinogens are a **partial agonist** at **postsynaptic serotonin receptors**, such as $5HT_{2A}$

-agonist action at $5HT_{2C}$ receptors is responsible for **hallucinogenic effects**

-stimulation of $5HT_{2C}$ receptors may promote one type of psychotic activity (LSD hallucinosis) while stimulation of $5HT_{2A}$ receptors may suppress another type (PCP psychosis)

-may explain PCP exacerbation of schizophrenic psychosis while LSD does not

M

Major Depressive Disorder, prepubertal child and adolescent
-likely to be manifest by **somatic** complaints, **psychomotor agitation**, and **mood-congruent hallucinations**

-anhedonia is frequent; anhedonia, hopelessness, psychomotor retardation, and delusions are more common in adolescent and adult major depressive episodes

-adults have more problems w/ sleep and appetite *than* depressed children and adolescents

-in **adolescence**, negativistic or frankly antisocial behavior and use of alcohol or illicit substances can occur; may justify additional diagnoses of oppositional defiant disorder, conduct disorder, and substance abuse or dependence

-feelings of **restlessness**, **grouchiness**, **aggression**, **sulkiness**, reluctance to cooperate in family ventures, **withdrawal from social activities**, and a desire to leave home are all common in adolescent depression

-**school difficulties** are likely; adolescents may be inattentive to personal appearance and show increased emotionality, w/ particular sensitivity to rejection in love relationships

Major Depressive Disorder; epidemiology, leading cause of disability
-**leading cause of disability** in U.S. for ages **15-44 yrs**

-affects ~**14.8 million** U.S. adults, or ~6.7% of U.S. age 18 and older in a given year

-**median** age at onset is **32 yrs**; more prevalent in **women** than in men

Malpractice 4 Ds
-a tort, or civil wrong

4 basic elements to prove medical malpractice:

-**duty** *of care*; a doctor-patient relationship existed

-**deviation** *from the standard of care*

-**damage** (*or harm*) to the patient

-**direct** *causation* of damage from deviation from standard of care

ALL 4 elements *must* **be present** for finding of liability

MAOI and meperidine, drug interaction

-extensive inhibition of MAO enzymes by MAOIs raises potential for drug interactions

-many over-the-counter medications can interact w/ MAOIs; include **cough syrups containing sympathomimetic agents**, which can precipitate **hypertensive crisis**

-caution should be taken w/use of MAOIs in patients who need surgery; interactions include those w/ narcotic drugs, *especially* **meperidine**

-meperidine administered w/ MAOIs can produce a syndrome characterized by **coma**, **hyperpyrexia**, and **HTN**; this has **primarily been reported w/ phenelzine**; also reported w/ tranylcypromine

-syndrome is most likely to occur w/ meperidine and it may be related to meperidine's serotonergic properties

-similar reactions have not been reported to any significant extent w/ other narcotic analgesics such as morphine and codeine

-current opinion favors the use of morphine or fentanyl when intra- or postoperative narcotics are needed in patients taking MAOIs

-in general, direct sympathomimetic amine–MAOI interactions do not appear to produce significant cardiovascular problems

-low incidence of hypertensive episodes in presence of indirect sympathomimetics; direct-acting compound is preferable

-caution should be exercised when using MAOIs in patients w/ pheochromocytoma and cardiovascular, cerebrovascular, and hepatic dz

-phenelzine tablets contain **gluten**; should NOT be given to patients w/ celiac dz

Maple Syrup Urine Disease (MSUD)

-in untreated neonates is characterized by **maple syrup odor** in **cerumen** and **urine** at **12-24 hrs after birth**

-elevated plasma concentrations of branched-chain amino acids (BCAAs) (leucine, isoleucine, and valine) and allo-isoleucine

-additionally, **ketonuria**, **irritability**, and **poor feeding** by **age 2-3 days**

-deepening encephalopathy manifesting as **lethargy**, intermittent **apnea**, **opisthotonus**, and **stereotyped movements** such as "fencing" and "bicycling" by **age 4-5 days**

-**coma** and **central respiratory failure** that may occur by **age 7-10 days**

-Rarely, milder variants of MSUD can present as anorexia, poor growth, irritability, or developmental delays later in infancy or childhood (Chuang & Shih 2001)

-individuals w/ intermediate or intermittent forms of MSUD can experience severe metabolic intoxication and encephalopathy under sufficient catabolic stress

MCV and Nonspecific Biological Markers in Alcohol Use

-many lab tests have been used in evaluation of substance abuse, none is diagnostic

-most useful lab tests to confirm alcohol-abuse problems are gamma-glutamyl transpeptidase (**GGT**), mean corpuscular volume (**MCV**), and carbohydrate-deficient transferrin (**CDT**); are **nonspecific** but can add to the evidence of alcohol abuse

-urine tox screen is best test to confirm problems w/other drugs

-serum **GGT** determination is one of the most widely used laboratory tests; hepatic enzyme is elevated in patients who use alcohol excessively; has a **higher sensitivity** *than* specificity b/c other conditions, such as nonalcoholic liver dz, hyperthyroidism, and use of anticonvulsants, can elevate GGT levels

-**MCV** also used as **marker of heavy alcohol consumption**; tends to be **less sensitive** *than* measurement of GGT level, but elevated MCV level combined w/ elevated GGT should raise suspicion about alcohol abuse

-**CDT** tests are available to **screen for excessive alcohol consumption**; has been estimated that 4-7 drinks per day for at least 1 week can significantly elevate CDT levels in patients w/alcoholism

MDMA mechanism of action, signs and symptoms

-affects many neurotransmitter systems; primarily **serotonergic** as an *indirect* **serotonergic agonist**

-**effects** and **side effects** are a result of *flooding* of **serotonin system**

-onset of effect begins **~20-40 min after ingestion** and is experience as a **sudden, amphetamine-like "rush"**

-**nausea**, usually mild, but sometimes severe enough to cause vomiting

-**plateau** stage of drug effects last **3-4 hours**

-principal desired effect, according to most users, is profound **feeling of relatedness** to the rest of the world

-in general, people taking the drug appear to be less aggressive and less impulsive

-drastically **altered perception of time** and a decreased inclination to perform mental and physical tasks

-although desire for sex can increase, **ability to achieve arousal and orgasm is greatly diminished** in both men and women

-may experience mild psychomotor **restlessness, bruxism, trismus, anorexia, diaphoresis, hot flashes, tremor** and **piloerection**

-common after effects can be pronounced, sometimes lasting 24 hours or more; most dramatic hangover effect is severe anhedonia; share many similarities w/amphetamine withdrawal

-can experience lethargy, anorexia, decreased motivation, sleepiness, depressed mood and fatigue, occasionally lasting for days

-in a few instances, more severe effects; including altered mental status, convulsions, hypo or hyperthermia, severe changes in BP, tachycardia, coagulopathy, acute renal failure, hepatotoxicity, and death

-tx of intoxication; keep patient hydrated

-acute MDMA reactions resemble combination of serotonin syndrome and NMS, uncommon but potentially fatal occurrence

Meaningful life, Integrity versus Despair (~ 60 yrs to Death)

-in *Identity: Youth and Crisis*, Erikson defined integrity as "the **acceptance of one's one and only life cycle** and of the persons who have become significant to it as something that had to be and that, by necessity, permitted of no substitutions."

-individual **relinquishes wish that important persons in his life had been different** and is **able to love in a more meaningful way**—one that reflects **accepting responsibility for one's own life**

-individual in possession of virtue of wisdom and sense of integrity has room to **tolerate proximity of death** and to achieve what Erikson termed in *Identity: Youth and Crisis* a "detached yet active concern with life."

-Erikson underlined social context for final stage of growth; in *Childhood and Society*, he wrote, "The style of integrity developed by his culture or civilization thus becomes the 'patrimony' of his soul.... In such final consolidation, death loses its sting."

-when attempt to attain integrity has failed, individual may become deeply disgusted w/ external world and contemptuous of persons as well as institutions

-Erikson wrote in *Childhood and Society* that such disgust masks fear of death and sense of despair that "time is now short, too short for the attempt to start another life and to try out alternate roads to integrity."

-looking back on the eight ages of man, he noted relation b/w adult integrity and infantile trust, "Healthy children will not fear life if their elders have integrity enough not to fear death."

Methadone, medication interactions

-**carbamazepine**, **phenytoin**, **rifampin**, **efavirenz**, **nevirapine**, **phenobarbital**, and *possibly* **risperidone** *induce* cytochrome P450 hepatic enzymes and *increase* methadone metabolism; *may* lead to **withdrawal sxs**

-**risperidone** *may* also precipitate **opioid withdrawal**, through **interference w/ methadone absorption** or a direct **effect on opioid receptors**

-**ciprofloxacin**, **fluoxetine**, **fluvoxamine**, **fluconazole** *inhibit* cytochrome P450 enzymes and *inhibit* methadone metabolism; *may* lead to **sedation**, **confusion**, or **respiratory depression**

-methadone also affects the metabolism of other medications (e.g., *increases* plasma levels of **desipramine**, **amitriptyline**, and **zidovudine** and may increase dose-related toxicity of these medications)

-methadone interactions w/ antiretroviral medications are of particular interest because of high prevalence of HIV infection among injection drug users

-nelfinavir causes substantial decreases (40%) in plasma methadone; can be a/w withdrawal sxs

-methadone-induced decreased GI motility, however, leads to increased GI degradation of stavudine and didanosine and significant decreases in plasma concentrations of these medications

Metoclopramide, acute dystonic reaction

-occur in 0.5-1% of patients given **metoclopramide** or **prochlorperazine**

-**up to 1/3** of acutely psychotic patients will have some sort of **drug-induced movement disorder** w/in **first few days of tx** w/ a **typical antipsychotic**

-**younger men** are at *higher* risk of acute EPS

-case reports of oculogyric crises from other classes of drugs, including **H$_2$ antagonists**, **erythromycin** and **antihistamines**; majority of acute dystonic reactions are from antiemetic or antipsychotic

MI mortality, effects of depression

-**major depression**; **significant predictor of mortality** *after* **acute MI**

-equal to the effect of predictors such as hx of MI or indexes of cardiac function

-in cohort of 3,000 individuals ages 55-85 for 4 years, **major depression tripled relative risk of cardiac mortality** in those **w/o heart dz** and **quadrupled** it in those **who did have cardiac dz**

-patients hospitalized for unstable angina who also had depressive sxs were four times more likely to have MI or die in following year than were those w/o depression (after adjusting for other factors)

Middle cerebral artery lesions

-occlusion occurs at stem of middle cerebral or at one of the 2 divisions of the artery in the sylvian sulcus

Superior Division

-**most common cause** of occlusion of superior division of MCA is an **embolus** (superior division of MCA supplies rolandic and prerolandic areas)

-sensory and motor deficits on contralateral face and arm > leg

-**head** and **eyes** *deviated* **toward side of infarct**

-w/ **left**-side lesion (***dominant* hemisphere**); **global** aphasia initially, then turns into **Broca's aphasia** (motor speech disorder)

-**right**-side lesion (*nondominant* **hemisphere**); deficits on **spatial** perception, **hemineglect**, **constructional** apraxia, **dressing** apraxia

-muscle tone usually decreased initially and gradually increases over days or weeks to spasticity

-transient loss of consciousness is uncommon

Inferior division (lateral temporal and inferior parietal lobes)

-w/ lesion on either side; superior quadrantanopia or homonymous hemianopsia

-left-side lesion, Wernicke's aphasia

-right-side lesion, left visual neglect

Mild Mental Retardation (MR), academic level of function in late teens
-roughly equivalent to what used to be referred to as educational category of **"educable"**

-constitutes **largest segment (~85%)** of **MR**

-typically develop social and communication skills during preschool years (ages 0-5 yrs)

-minimal impairment in sensorimotor areas

-often are not distinguishable from children w/o MR until later age

-**late teens** can acquire academic skills up to ~ **sixth-grade level**

-**adult years** usually achieve social and vocational skills adequate for **minimum self-support**, but *may* **need** **supervision**, **guidance**, and **assistance**, especially when under unusual social or economic stress

-w/ appropriate supports, individuals w/ Mild MR can usually live successfully in the community, either independently or in supervised settings

Minnesota Multiphasic Personality Inventory (MMPI)
-developed in 1940s by J. Charnley McKinley, psychiatrist, and Starke R. Hathaway, psychologist

-items were generated from lists of psychiatric sxs and complaints found in current textbooks of psychiatry and previously constructed personality inventories

-used method of contrasting criterion groups to construct several psychopathological scales

-consists of 10 clinical scales: Hypochondriasis (Scale 1), Depression (Scale 2), Hysteria (Scale 3), Psychopathic Deviance (Scale 4), Masculinity–Femininity (Scale 5), Paranoia (Scale 6), Psychasthenia (Scale 7), Schizophrenia (Scale 8), and Mania (Scale 9), Social Introversion (Scale 10)

-items were worded so that persons w/ elementary school education could take the test

-norms established for determining degree of disturbance typical of psychopathological groups

-validity scales developed to assess test-taking attitudes of patient

-focused on assessment of defensiveness or minimizing sxs and problems (faking good) and maximizing or exaggerating problems (faking bad)

-MMPI revised and restandardized as MMPI-2

-revisions include deletion of objectionable items and rewording of other items to reflect more modern language usage, as well as the addition of several *new* **items** focusing on **suicide**, **drug and alcohol abuse**, **Type A behavior**, **interpersonal relations**, and **tx compliance**

-**restandardization of norms** based on randomly solicited national sample of 1,138 males and 1,462 females; **limitation** includes *not* accounting for **religion** and **race** in normative data

Modeling, behavior therapy

-patients **learn new behavior** by **imitation**, primarily by **observation**, w/o having to perform behavior until they feel ready

-irrational fears *can* be **unlearned by observing a fearless model** confront feared object acquired by learning

-technique has been useful w/ phobic children who are placed w/ other children of their own age and sex who approach the feared object or situation

-therapist may describe the feared activity in a calm manner or act out the process of mastering the feared activity

-**hierarchy of activities** may be established, w/ least anxiety-provoking activity being dealt w/ first

-participant-modeling technique has been used successfully w/ agoraphobia by having a therapist accompany a patient into feared situation; behavior rehearsal, is a variant of the procedure where real-life problems are acted out under therapist's observation or direction

Motivational interviewing, patient resistant to treatment

-first developed for use w/ individuals w/ substance use disorders by William R. **Miller** and Stephen **Rollnick** (1991)

-**patient-centered**, **directive** method for **enhancing intrinsic motivation** to **change** by **exploring** and **resolving ambivalence**

-focuses on individual's **present interests** and **difficulties** and tries to resolve ambivalence by eliciting and selectively reinforcing 'change talk,' to move towards change

-change is thought to arise through its **relevance to individual's own values** and **concerns**

-technique has continued to develop and is now used for a variety of clinical problems and lifestyle changes

-research supports efficacy of motivational interviewing techniques for substance use d/o, as well as for individuals w/ diabetes, HTN, dual dx, and bulimia

Multiaxial system, DSM-III

-introduced in U.S. in mid-1970s; widely regarded as one of the most important contributions of **DSM-III**, published in 1980

-patient is **evaluated** in terms of **several different domains of information** that are assumed to be of high clinical value

Multiple Sclerosis, Dementia

Multiple sclerosis, treatment of acute exacerbation with methylprednisolone
-corticosteroids are often used to improve rate of recovery from acute exacerbation in MS

-6 trials contributed to review w/ total of 377 participants (199 treatment, 178 placebo) were randomized; drugs analyzed were **methylprednisolone** (**MP**) (4 trials, 140 participants) and ACTH (2 trials, 237 participants)

-MP or ACTH showed protective effect against MS getting worse or stable w/in first 5 weeks of tx (odds ratio 0.37, 95% CI 0.24 to 0.57) w/ some but non-significant greater effect for MP and IV administration

-short (5 days) or long (15 days) duration of tx w/ MP did not show any significant difference; no data are available beyond 1 year of f/u to indicate whether steroids or ACTH have any effect on long-term progression

-1 study reported that short term tx w/high dose IV MP was NOT attended by adverse events; GI sxs and psychic disorders were significantly more common in oral, high-dose MP than in placebo group; weight gain and edema were significantly more frequent in ACTH group than controls

-evidenced *favored* **methylprednisolone** for **acute exacerbation in MS patients**; data are insufficient to reliably estimate effect of corticosteroids on prevention of new exacerbations and reduction of long-term disability

Myasthenia gravis, diagnosis
-clinical dx, confirmed by **positive Tensilon** (edrophonium) **test**, by detection of **serum ACh receptor antibodies**, or by obtaining **EMG**

-**fluctuating**, *asymmetric* **weakness of the extraocular, facial**, and **bulbar muscles**

-repeated activities weaken muscles; sxs often **first develop *only* in late afternoon** or **early evening**

- **~90%**, typically **young women** or **older men**, develop **diplopia** or **ptosis** as their *first* **symptom**

-severe cases cause respiratory distress, quadriplegia, and inability to speak (anarthria)

M'Naughten rule, insanity defense

-precedent for determining legal responsibility established in 1843 in British courts; known commonly as the ***right-wrong*** test

-until recently, has determined criminal responsibility in most of the U.S.

-holds that persons are ***not* guilty by reason of insanity** *if* they labored under **mental dz** such that they were **unaware of the nature**, **quality**, and **consequences** of their acts *or* if they were **incapable of realizing** that their acts were wrong

-to absolve persons from punishment, a **delusion used as evidence** *must* be one that, ***if* true, would be an adequate defense**

-if the delusional idea does not justify the crime, such persons are presumably held responsible, guilty, and punishable

-rule derives from famous M'Naghten case of 1843; Daniel M'Naghten, private secretary of Robert Peel, M'Naghten had been suffering from delusions of persecution for several years and murdered Edward Drummond

-question is whether the defendant ***understood the nature and the quality* of the act** and whether the defendant **knew the difference b/w right and wrong *w/ respect to the act***

-specifically, whether the defendant knew the act was wrong or perhaps thought the act was correct, a delusion causing the defendant to act in legitimate self-defense

N

Narcissism
-in psychoanalytic theory, divided into **primary** and **secondary** types

-*primary* narcissism, early **infantile phase of object relationship** development

-child has **not differentiated** the **self from outside world**

-all sources of pleasure are unrealistically recognized as **coming from w/in the self**, giving the child a **false sense of omnipotence**

-*secondary* narcissism, when the libido, once **attached to external love objects**, is **redirected back to the self**

Narcissistic vulnerability, empathy from caregivers
-**Self** theorists believe **parental feedback** *lacking* **in empathy and attention** may eventually undermine inherently healthy narcissistic potential and lead a **child to remain fixated at an infantile**, **self-centered**, **"grandiose" stage of development**, constantly craving attention (Watson et al. 1993)

-**Kohut** (1971), overt narcissism results when **rudimentary self formed in childhood** *fails* **to be integrated properly** w/ rest of the personality, owing to *inadequate* **mirroring** (i.e., encouraging praise and expressions of acceptance that inform the child it is 'good') by the parent

-In an attempt to resume psychological growth process and fulfill unmet infantile needs, the **narcissistic** individual continues to express **grandiosity and exhibitionism** *into* adulthood

Negative symptoms, Schizophrenia
-thought to result from dysfunction of **dorsolateral prefrontal circuit**; underlies production of primary, enduring, negative or deficit sxs

-refer to clinical features resulting from *absence* **of normal mental functions**; long recognized as a core feature of this schizophrenia

-include deficits in **affective**, **social**, and **cognitive** realms

-once acute psychotic state is stabilized w/ tx, negative sxs *may* **be a stronger indicator of long-term disability**

Affective Deficits

-*blunting of affect* is a term describing decrease in amount and range of affective expressivity; refers to facial expressions in which normal expressions a/w emotional states are diminished or absent

-related descriptors are flat and constricted affect; defined as total absence of, and a moderate decrease in, affective expressivity, respectively

-once thought that these deficits reflected a fundamental abnormality in experiencing of emotions, particularly positive emotions or anhedonia; recent research reports that patients may experience equivalent levels of pleasure

-some research points to possibility that patients w/predominance of paranoid delusions may have heightened sensitivity to negative or threatening situations

-another common affective deficit is apathy, or apparent indifference to the consequences of his or her own or others' actions and decisions; can manifest as lack of motivation to initiate or maintain activity

Social Deficits

-increasingly recognized as important aspect; **social withdrawal**, little interest in participating in social events and interacting w/people

-often describe not needing to spend much time w/ other people and preferring to be by themselves; decreased social drive, do not derive pleasure from social interactions

Cognitive Deficits

-*alogia* or **poverty of speech** describes significant decrease in amount of unprompted speech given by a patient

-poverty of speech, give very short and unelaborated responses to questions; interviewer has to guide patient w/ numerous explicit questions to obtain responses w/sufficient detail

Neural tube defect, valproic acid

-prenatal exposure to valproate has been a/w numerous congenital malformations, including neural tube defects

-also a/w craniofacial anomalies, including craniosynostosis; limb abnormalities; and cardiovascular anomalies

-valproate **exposure *prior* to neural tube closure**, during **4th week of gestation**, **1%–2% risk** for spina bifida, **10-20 times *greater*** than prevalence in general population

-one meta-analysis placed risk for neural tube defects at 3.8%, w/particular vulnerability for infants of women whose **daily dose > 1,000 mg**, other studies support dose–response relationship w/ some recommending daily dose not to exceed 1,000 mg and maternal serum concentrations ***not exceed* max of 70 mcg/mL** to reduce risk for malformations

-*fetal valproate syndrome* initially reported by Di Liberti et al. (1984); stereotypical facial features such as bifrontal narrowing, midface hypoplasia, broad nasal bridge, short nose w/ anteverted nares, epicanthal folds, micrognathia, shallow philtrum, thin upper lip, and thick lower lip

-valproate's antagonistic effect on folate may also underlie full spectrum of fetal valproate syndrome

Neuroleptic malignant syndrome

-**potentially life-threatening** complication of antipsychotic use

-1% of all psychiatric admissions in patients treated w/ neuroleptics

-range 0.07% to 2.4% reported

-criteria for dx of NMS have fluctuated from article to article

-general agreement: **hyperthermia**, *severe* **EPS**, and **autonomic dysfunction**

-misdiagnosis can obviously occur but **severe muscle rigidity** often seen in NMS is rare feature of incidental infection

-serum CK levels can be increased by IM injections or by violent physical struggling; rarely >1,000 IU/mL

-neuroleptics can affect temperature-regulating brain centers; can be a/w heatstroke, particularly in hot weather or in hot seclusion rooms, in the absence of other manifestations of NMS

-neuroleptic-induced catatonia can occur in absence of fever

-NMS usually develops **over 1-3 days** in patients taking antipsychotics

-*many* **cases develop in first week**; *most* **w/in first month of tx** w/ antipsychotics

-weak evidence that concomitant tx w/ lithium may predispose patients to develop NMS

-NMS observed w/ all widely used neuroleptics; thioridazine underrepresented

-depot neuroleptics do NOT seem to be more likely to cause NMS; prolonged duration of action will make syndrome last about twice as long (Glazer and Kane 1992)

-best tx is *early* **identification**, **stopping** neuroleptics, rapid transfer to ICU in moderate to severe cases

-**dopamine agonist** bromocriptine 5 mg every 4 hrs, can often relieve muscle rigidity and reduce fever

-dantrolene is used in ICUs to reduce muscle spasm

-anticholinergic antiparkinsonian drugs are probably NOT helpful

-symptomatic tx (e.g., cooling the body) is helpful

-syndrome can recur after it appears to have been brought under control, so patients should be observed carefully for 1 month after condition is first noted

-neuroleptics should be avoided during that period

-ECT can be used successfully in treating persistently manic patients who have recently experienced an episode of NMS

-can restart neuroleptics cautiously at much lower dosages w/o recurrence of NMS

-not clear whether thioridazine is safer than one-quarter dosage of the original offending medication

-avoid depot antipsychotics in patients w/ hx of NMS

Neuropsychiatric manifestations of multiple sclerosis

-**40-60%** complain of **memory problems**; a/w plaque formation in temporal lobe and diencephalic areas

- ~25% develop euphoria that is *not* hypomania but different than premorbid mood

-25-50% develop **depression** a/w *higher* rate suicide

-20-40% develop **personality changes**; irritability and apathy are common

Nicotine dependence, sustained-release bupropion

-phenylaminoketone, atypical antidepressant agent bupropion

-in **sustained-release** (SR) formulation is non-nicotine, **first-line pharmacological tx for nicotine-dependent smokers** who want to quit smoking

-exact mechanism of action in tx of nicotine dependence is unclear, but likely to involve **dopamine** and **norepinephrine reuptake blockade**, as well as *antagonism* of **high-affinity nAChRs**

-goals of bupropion therapy are 1) smoking cessation, 2) reduction of nicotine craving and withdrawal sxs, and 3) prevention of cessation-induced weight gain

-target dose in nicotine dependence is 300 mg/day (150 mg, two times a day)

-typically started 7 days prior to target quit date at 150 mg/day; then increased to 150 mg 2 times a day after 3-4 days

-main contraindication for use of bupropion is past hx of seizures of any etiology; rates of de novo seizures are low w/ bupropion (<0.5%), at doses of 300 mg/day or less; observed when daily dosing exceeds 450 mg

Nonmaleficence

-modern term for old, rule of **primum non nocere (first, do no harm)**

-in medical ethics, *harm* is defined broadly, including **killing**, causing **physical or emotional suffering**, or **depriving** others of beneficial things

Number Needed to Treat (NNT)

-number of patients who need to be treated **in order to *prevent* one additional bad outcome** or to **produce one additional positive outcome**

-NNT is the **reciprocal of the Absolute Risk Reduction** (ARR),

1/(probability of control - probability of intervention)

-*effective* interventions have a *low* NNT

O

Object constancy
-fourth subphase of **separation-individuation** phase (third phase of infantile development in ego psychology)

-takes place in the **third year of life** and refers to the *integration* **of the good and bad aspects of the internalized images** of both the mother and the child's self

-considered *necessary* for later development of **stable and mature interpersonal relationships**

Obsessive-Compulsive Disorder, exposure and response prevention
-effective **behavior therapy** consists of **exposure** *in vivo* and **ritual prevention**

-when systematically applied lead to habituation of anxiety a/w obsessions so rituals are no longer needed to reduce anxiety

-rituals are performed to temporarily reduce discomfort and compulsion to ritualize

-ritual prevention is effective in reducing urge and discomfort but requires longer time to achieve reductions; learned through process of habituation when repeated through systematic exposure and ritual prevention homework assignments

- ~25% of OCD patients referred for behavior therapy decline or are noncompliant

-64% of patients who completed at least one E&RP session using computer-guided program in self-help homework exposure and ritual prevention was as helpful as 12 hrs of clinician-directed E&RP

Obsessive-Compulsive Disorder, SSRI implementation
-data suggest *higher* **SSRI doses** produce somewhat *higher* **response rate** and somewhat greater magnitude of **symptom relief**

-among nonresponders, **raising the dose of an SSRI** is a/w **enhanced response**

-literature does not allow specification of chance of response as function of number of previously failed adequate SRI trials

-clinical trial data are limited by differences in number of failed trials in patients included in a given study; absence of information about number of failed adequate trials; differences in definition of "failed," and by small, highly selected samples

-clinical experience suggests patients who do not respond to one SRI may still respond well to another

-w/ SRIs, response rates to second trial are close to 50% but may fall off as number of failed adequate trials increases

-switch to venlafaxine at 225-350 mg/day is also supported by active-comparator trials and open-label studies

Obsessive-Compulsive Disorder and Tourette's Disorder
-obsessive-compulsive d/o and Tourette's syndrome **frequently co-occur**

- ~90% of individuals w/ Tourette's d/o have compulsive sxs

-as many as **2/3 of individuals w/ Tourette's meet criteria for OCD**

-incidence of **Tourette's d/o in patients w/ OCD is 5-7%**

-20-30% of patients w/OCD have a hx of tics

Operant conditioning, extinction
-**B. F. Skinner** theory of learning and behavior known as operant conditioning

-in operant conditioning, person or animal is *active* (unlike classical conditioning) and **behaves in a way that produces a reward**; thus **learning** occurs as a **consequence of action**

-related to trial-and-error learning; person or animal attempts to solve problem by trying different actions until one proves successful

-behavior is **followed by a consequence** which **modifies tendency to repeat** behavior in future

-behavior **followed by reinforcing stimulus** results in *increased* **probability** of that **behavior occurring** in future

-*extinction* occurs when a **behavior is** *no longer* **reinforced**; *decreased* probability that a desired behavior will occur in the future **w/o reinforcement**

Overvalued idea

-**false** or **unreasonable belief or idea** that is **sustained** beyond the bounds of reason

-NOT ordinarily accepted by the person's culture or subculture

-it is held w/ **less intensity or duration than a delusion**, but is usually a/w mental illness

-when challenged, person is able to acknowledge may not be true

P

Pain syndromes, suicide risk
-literature has shown *chronic* pain conditions to be a/w *higher* rates of **suicidal ideation**, **suicide attempts**, and **completed suicides**

-data are *strongest* for **migraine** and suicidal ideation and suicide attempts

-among chronic pain patients, **abdominal pain** was a/w 5.5-fold increase in suicidal ideation and 4.2-fold increase in suicide attempts

-neuropathic pain was a/w reduced risk of suicidal ideation and suicide attempts

-*lack* of strong association b/w suicidal ideation and pain duration, pain severity, and depression severity

-limitations of studies on chronic pain and suicide risk; majority of previous studies have used treatment-seeking samples, studies have not examined whether there is differential relationship w/ suicidal ideation and suicide attempts across pain syndromes

Pain, treatment w/ transcutaneous electrical nerve stimulation (TENS)
-**proposed mechanisms** for neuromodulation:

Presynaptic inhibition in the dorsal horn of the spinal cord

Endogenous pain control via endorphins, enkephalins, and dynorphins

Direct inhibition of abnormally excited nerve

Restoration of afferent input

-literature on effectiveness; wide range of outcomes

-overall consensus favoring use of TENS; provides initial relief of pain 70-80% of patients, success rate decreases after few months or longer, 20-30%

-trial of TENS for at least 1 hr should be given to confirm potential benefit

Indications

Neurogenic pain, **peripheral neuralgia**

Musculoskeletal pain, ***most* effective** for **mild to moderate levels of pain**, American Academy of Neurology recommended against use for tx of chronic LBP

Visceral pain and dysmenorrhea

Diabetic neuropathy

Contraindications

-patients w/ pacemaker, especially demand type

-during pregnancy, may induce premature labor

-NOT applied over carotid sinuses, risk of vasovagal reflex and acute hypotension

-NOT over anterior neck, risk of laryngospasm d/t laryngeal muscle contraction

-NOT placed over area of sensory impairment (nerve lesions, neuropathies), risk of burns

-used cautiously w/ spinal cord stimulator or intrathecal pump

Panic attacks, symptoms
-usually last from 5-20 minutes, rarely as long as 1 hr

-**sudden onset** of overwhelming **fear**, **terror**, **apprehension**, and sense of **impending doom**

-associated sxs include: dyspnea, palpitations, chest pain or discomfort, choking or smothering sensations, dizziness or feeling unsteady, derealization and/or depersonalization, paresthesias, hot and cold flashes, sweating, faintness, trembling and shaking, and fear of dying, going crazy, or losing control of oneself

-physical sensations, massive overstimulation of autonomic nervous system

-can progress until level of fearfulness and autonomic hyperactivity in interval b/w panic attacks almost approximates level during a panic attack

-**hyperventilation**, considered the **cardinal symptom of panic**, may be **central feature in the pathophysiology** of panic attacks and panic d/o

-individuals w/ panic d/o shown to be chronic hyperventilators; acutely hyperventilate during spontaneous and induced panic, induces hypocapnia and alkalosis, leading to decreased cerebral blood flow and to dizziness, confusion, and derealization characteristic of panic attacks

-signs and sxs of hyperventilation seem to disappear w/ successful tx

-behavioral breathing retraining may decrease frequency of panic attacks, possibly by dampening ventilatory overreaction

Panic Disorder, psychoanalytic theories

-conceptualize panic attacks as arising from unsuccessful defense against anxiety-provoking impulses

-previously mild signal anxiety becomes overwhelming feeling of apprehension, complete w/ somatic sxs

-emphasize **loss of a parent in childhood** and **hx of separation anxiety d/o**; being alone in public places revives childhood anxiety about being abandoned

-defense mechanisms used include repression, displacement, avoidance, and symbolization

-traumatic separations during childhood can affect children's developing nervous systems in such a manner that they become susceptible to anxieties in adulthood

-many patients describe panic attacks as coming out of the blue; psychodynamic exploration frequently reveals a clear psychological trigger for panic attack

-patients w/ panic d/o have **higher incidence of stressful life events** (particularly loss) than control subjects **in months before onset** of panic d/o

-typically experience **greater distress about life events** *than* control subjects

-research indicates that cause of panic attacks is likely to involve unconscious meaning of stressful events and that pathogenesis of panic attacks may be related to neurophysiological factors triggered by psychological reactions

parens patriae

-"father of his country"

-in U.S. common law, *allows* state to **act for people** who are **mentally ill** and for **minors**

Pediatric Mood Disorders, clinical presentation
Depressive Disorders

-prevalence of up to 14% in adolescents

-children do not seek help easily, contributing to previous underestimate of prevalence

-presentation may differ from adults; depressed children *may* **show irritability rather than depressed mood**

-younger children may have more appetite changes and delusional thinking

-associated features include low self-esteem, negative cognitions, and behavioral difficulties

-essential to screen for comorbid conditions; learning disability, ADHD, disruptive behavior disorders, and anxiety d/o

-children w/ chronic medical problems, including diabetes, asthma, and epilepsy, also have a high rate of depression

Bipolar Disorder

-prevalence of bipolar disorder in children and adolescents is **~1%**

-bipolar d/o is **difficult to dx** in children **< 10 yrs**

-characterized by irritability, cyclical mood changes, and associated ADHD

-clinical course may follow more chronic, undulating pattern, w/ fewer discrete mood episodes

-adolescents are more likely to present w/ typical features of bipolar d/o

-differential dx includes ADHD; presence of **elevated mood**, **grandiosity**, **flight of ideas**, and *decreased need for sleep* are features unique to bipolar disorder

Pernicious anemia, neuropsychiatric symptoms

-chronic illness caused by **impaired absorption of vitamin B12** because of a lack of intrinsic factor (IF) in gastric secretions

-adult pernicious anemia usually occurs at age **40-70 yrs**; among white patients, mean age of onset is 60 yrs; occurs at younger age in black people (mean age 50 yrs)

-congenital pernicious anemia is usually manifested in children < 2 yrs

-**onset** is *insidious* and *vague*; classic triad of **weakness**, **sore tongue**, and **paresthesias**

-CNS sxs include **somnolence**, **dementia**, *psychotic* **depression**, and occasionally frank **psychosis**; may demonstrate **combined system dz** (posterolateral column), paresthesias in fingers and toes or difficulty w/ gait and balance, loss of position sense and loss of vibratory sense for a 256-Hz

-medical attention is usually sought because of sxs suggestive of cardiac, renal, GU, GI, infectious, mental, or neurological disorders

-often **anemic w/ macrocytic cellular indices**

Pervasive Developmental Disorder Not Otherwise Specified

-child w/ **severe** and **pervasive impairment** in development of **reciprocal social interaction** or **verbal and nonverbal communication**, or **stereotyped behavior**, **interests**, and **activities** are present

-does **NOT** meet criteria for any of the more specific pervasive developmental disorders, Autistic D/O, Rett's D/O, Childhood Disintegrative D/O, Asperger's D/O

Piaget, intellectual development

-Piaget's interest in cognitive development came from training in natural sciences and interest in epistemology (study of knowledge)

-very interested in **knowledge** and *how* **children come to know their world**

-developed cognitive theory by actually observing children, including his own

-used standard questions or set of questions; followed **child's train of thought** and allowed questioning to be flexible

-believed children's spontaneous comments provided valuable clues to understanding their thinking

-NOT interested in a right or wrong answer, but rather what forms of logic and reasoning the child used

-concluded that intellectual development is result of the interaction of hereditary and environmental factors; as the child develops and constantly interacts w/ the world around him, knowledge is invented and reinvented

-theory of intellectual development is strongly grounded in biological sciences; cognitive growth as extension of biological growth and as being governed by same laws and principles

-argued that intellectual development controlled every other aspect of development (emotional, social, and moral)

Pituitary adenomas; mental, physical, visual abnormalities

-tx varies considerably from glioblastomas, astrocytomas, and meningiomas ('brain tumors')

-massive tumors produce extraordinary levels of hormone; expand out of the diaphragm sella and encroach on the adjacent temporal lobes and optic chiasm; **obstruct CSF flow through third ventricle**

-most tumors are **prolactinomas** (secretes prolactin and usually remains **microscopic**) or **chromophobe** (does NOT secrete prolactin and **typically grow large enough to exert pressure** on surrounding structures) adenomas

-upward pressure on diaphragm sellae usually causes:

Bitemporal and generalized **headache**; compress optic chiasm w/ **bitemporal superior quadrantanopia**; **bitemporal hemianopsia** w/ further enlargement

-*before* visual field defects, may insidiously cause **pituitary hormone insufficiency**:

Infertility, amenorrhea, decreased libido, and galactorrhea

-eventual **hormone failure**:

Lack of energy, apathy, and listlessness

-individual seems **depressed** *but* retains cognitive capacity

-less commonly, pituitary growths secrete growth hormone:

Acromegaly, or adrenocorticotropin (ACTH), can lead to Cushing's syndrome; can cause depression and psychosis

Play therapy, infants and young children
-child's developmental level of functioning is determined by combining observations made during interview w/ standardized developmental measures

-**observations of play** reveal a child's developmental level and reflect the child's **emotional state and preoccupations**

-examiner can interact w/ infant age **18 mos or younger** in playful manner by using such games as **peek-a-boo**

-**18 mos to 3 yrs**; can be **observed in a playroom**

-**2 yrs or older** *may* exhibit **symbolic play w/ toys**, revealing more than through conversation

-use of **puppets and dolls w/ children < 6 yrs** is often an effective way to elicit information, *especially* if **questions are directed to the dolls**, rather than to the child

Play, developmental landmarks
-begin to distinguish reality from fantasy, reflected through play

-pretend games are popular and help test real-life situations in playful manner

-dramatic play in which children act out a role is common; 1:1 play relationships advance to complicated patterns

-children's play behavior reflects level of social development

-**2½-3 yrs**, commonly engage in **parallel play, solitary play** *alongside* another child **w/ no interaction**

-by **3 yrs**, play is often **associative**; playing **w/ same toys in pairs** or in **small groups**, but *still* **w/ no real interaction**

-by **4 yrs**, usually able to **share and engage in cooperative play**, **real interactions** and **taking turns** become possible

-**3-6 yrs**, growth can be traced *through* **drawings**

-child's first drawing of human being is circular line w/ marks for mouth, nose, and eyes

-ears and hair are added later; arms and stick-like fingers appear next; and then legs appear; *last* to appear is torso in proportion to rest of body

-intelligent children can deal w/ details in their art

-drawings express creativity throughout development; representational and formal in early childhood; use of perspective in middle childhood; abstract and affect laden in adolescence

-drawings also reflect children's body image concepts, sexual and aggressive impulses

Power Analysis

-analytical method for estimating the **sample size required** to **detect statistical effects** of a **defined size** for **variables w/ known variances**

-choice of the **outcome measure** *must be in accordance* w/ choice of the **analytic procedure**

-better selection of the outcome measure has a major impact on the study's power and necessary sample size

Pramipexole, side effects

-stimulates dopamine receptors in corpus striatum

-dopamine agonists, long used in treating Parkinson's dz and effective in relieving sxs of restless legs syndrome

-case reports have begun to appear linking **dopamine agonists w/ new-onset compulsions** in RLS patients

-survey study at a movement-disorders clinic found 10% of respondents w/ RLS on dopamine agonists (8/77) reported either **increased gambling** (5/70) or **increased libido** (4/77), w/ 1 patient reporting both (Driver-Dunckley et al. 2003)

-rates of clearly pathological behaviors, behaviors affecting social or occupational functioning, *as high as* **13%** have been **reported w/ therapeutic dopamine agonist doses**, defined as >2 mg pramipexole or 6 mg ropinirole daily (Bostwick et al. 2009)

Premenstrual Dysphoric Disorder, treatment with fluoxetine

-**serotonergic system** has close relationship w/ gonadal hormones; identified as most plausible target for intervention

-several RCTs in women w/ PMDD have clearly demonstrated SSRIs have excellent efficacy and minimal adverse effects

-several studies indicate that **intermittent tx w/ SSRIs** limited to premenstrual phase is **equally effective**

-Cochrane Systematic Review demonstrated **ALL SSRIs** (fluoxetine, paroxetine, sertraline, fluvoxamine, citalopram, and clomipramine) were **effective** in *reducing* premenstrual sxs

-**fluoxetine** (first approved), **sertraline**, and **paroxetine controlled release** are **FDA-approved** SSRIs for PMDD

-large, randomized, controlled study reported fluoxetine superior to placebo in reducing sxs of tension, irritability, and dysphoria; less effective in controlling physical sxs

-**fluoxetine** at **20 or 60 mg/d** through 6 menstrual cycles improved mood sxs in 53% of cycles compared w/ improvement in 28% of cycles w/ placebo

-women who received **60 mg** of fluoxetine per day reported significantly *more* **side effects** than those who received 20 mg per day or placebo

-common adverse effects include nausea, headache, weight gain, rash, fatigue, insomnia, anxiety, nervousness, and somnolence

-long-term study reported sexual dysfunction, decreased libido and anorgasmia, as most common adverse effect (17% of patients)

Preoperational Phase (2-7 yrs), cognitive development

-one of **Piaget's 4 stages of cognitive development**: sensorimotor, preoperational thought, concrete operations, and formal operations

-children **use symbols and language** > sensorimotor stage

-thinking and reasoning are intuitive; **learn w/o reasoning**

-unable to think logically or deductively, concepts are primitive

-events are not linked by logic, **no sense of cause and effect**

-can **name** objects but *not* **classes** of objects

-considered transition b/w completely autistic freudian unconscious and socialized adult thought

-cannot grasp sameness of object in different circumstances, same object in 3 locations is perceived as 3 different objects

-things are represented in terms of their function

-begin to use language and drawings in more elaborate ways

-cannot deal w/ moral dilemmas but have sense of what is good and bad

-**egocentric**, see themselves as center of the universe, limited point of view, unable to take role of another person

-use type of magical thinking, *phenomenalistic causality*, events that occur together are thought to cause one another

-use *animistic thinking*, endow physical events and objects w/ life-like psychological attributes, feelings and intentions

-**semiotic function** w/ symbolic gesture, or use of symbol or sign to stand for something else

Primary Gain

-patients achieve primary gain by **keeping internal conflicts *outside* their awareness**

-sxs have **symbolic value**; represent an **unconscious psychological conflict**

-clinical example is a patient that becomes enraged w/ his spouse and threatens to strike her; his arm becomes "limp" shortly after the argument and he presents w/ complaint of inability to move his arm

Projective Identification

-Klein defined as "a combination of **splitting off parts of the self** and **projecting them onto another person**," later describing it as "the feeling of identification with other people because one has attributed qualities or attributes of one's own to them"

-defensive mode evolving from **early infantile developmental stage** in which anxiety is **warded off by experiencing intolerable affects**, especially aggression, as if they **resided in a space external to the self**

-when interacting w/ another person, behavior toward the other is determined by our mental image of him or her; disavowed aspects of self and cherished aspects of self are projected

-our consequent behavior impinges on and affects that other person, but the person we are relating to exists only w/in our mind as a construct

-we never truly know the other person and what he or she feels; we can only approximate the actuality and subjectivity of the external object by drawing on our own experience and attempting to match it w/ what our senses are receiving from outside

-empathy is the highest-level transformation of projective identification

-a *hallmark* of defensive projective identification is the **sense of certainty that the subject has of the nature of the other** and *inflexibility* **of the subject's perceptions** regardless of what the other may be communicating that may differ from these perceptions

Prolactinemia associated with antipsychotics

-can result in reduced spermatogenesis, gynecomastia, loss of sexual desire, erectile failure in men

-amenorrhea, altered ovarian cycle, hirsutism, reduced sexual desire in women

-above effects result from high levels of prolactin combined w/decreased levels of FSH and LH

-*blockade* **of tuberoinfundibular tract** projecting to hypothalamus and pituitary gland results in multiple neuroendocrine side effects through pituitary gland

-**dopamine** is responsible for **tonic inhibition of prolactin release**

-prolactin release is no longer prevented w/ significant dopaminergic blockade of tuberoinfundibular tract; decrease in other pituitary influenced hormones requiring dopamine

Pruning, synaptic connections

-programmed elimination during development of neurons, synapses, axons, and other brain structures from the original number present at birth

-visual cortex neurons increase from birth to 3 yrs at which time they diminish in number

- ~**2x as many synapses** are present in certain parts of the cerebral cortex *during* **early postnatal life** *than* **during adulthood**

-**adolescence** is marked by **pruning of 1/2 of synaptic connections** seen at birth w/ decreased glucose and oxygen metabolism and decreased EEG amplitude

Psychotic Features, Major Depression

-presence of psychotic features, *reflects* **severe dz**

-*poor* **prognostic indicator**

-literature suggests distinct **differences in pathogenesis** b/w psychotic w/ nonpsychotic major depressive d/o

-**bipolar I d/o** is more common in **families w/ psychotic depression**

-psychotic sxs are often categorized as mood congruent or mood incongruent

-patients **w/ mood-incongruent** psychotic sxs *may* **have schizoaffective d/o or schizophrenia**

-poor prognosis for patients w/ mood disorders:

Long duration of episodes

Temporal dissociation b/w mood d/o and psychotic sxs

Poor premorbid hx of social adjustment

-presence of psychotic features has significant tx implications; *typically* require **antipsychotic drugs** in addition to antidepressants or mood stabilizers

-*may* need **ECT** for clinical improvement

Pulmonary Disease and Panic Disorder

-research has repeatedly demonstrated that **panic disorder** is **highly prevalent among patients w/ asthma** and other **chronic obstructive pulmonary dz**

-individuals **w/ panic d/o** have *higher* **lifetime prevalence of respiratory dz** *than* controls

-large-scale survey (Goodwin & Pine, 2002) found asthma, chronic bronchitis, and emphysema to be a/w an increased risk of panic

Radiculopathy, clinical signs and symptoms

-mostly seen in middle aged males, unless trauma

-**L4/5** and **L5/S1** disc protrusion ~**90% of cases**, each level affected equally; L3/4 disc accounts for remaining

-nerve roots exit through intervertebral foramen caudal to corresponding vertebral pedicle (L5 root exits at L5/S1 intervertebral foramen); majority of disc herniations are **posterolateral** and **compress the root** that exits at intervertebral foramen **below level of involved disc** (L5 root in L4/5)

-acute sxs often follow trauma or injury to disc w/ spinal strain

-acute low back pain; radiating pain, paresthesias, and motor weakness w/ nerve root compression

-severe bilateral root dysfunction may produce bowel and bladder incontinence and sexual dysfunction

-leg pain may present over hrs w/ paresthesias; in dermatomal fashion

-back pain thought to be secondary to activation of sinu-vertebral nerves to annulus, share a central pathway w/ nerve roots

-chronic sxs characterized by intermittent exacerbations of back ache, usually w/o leg pain initially, usually subsides w/ rest and conservative tx; leg pain may be as well localized as in acute state

-pain is aggravated by increased activities, bending forwards, coughing, sneezing, and straining w/ defecation; prolonged sitting increases intradiscal pressure and pain

-paraspinal muscles are often in spasm, particularly opposite side of leg pain, tender to palpation

-patient leans away from side of leg pain w/ hip and knee flexed to reduce leg pain

-spinal movements are restricted d/t pain; lateral bending towards side of leg pain closes intervertebral foramen, compresses nerve root and worsens pain

-pain exacerbated by straight leg raise and crossed straight leg (contra lateral leg) raising stretches sciatic nerve, L5, and S1 root

-neurological exam may detect motor, sensory, and reflex impairment, lower motor neuron

-**L5** radiculopathy may present w/ pain, and paresthesia/numbness along **posterolateral aspect of leg down to great toe**; **weakness of extensor hallusis longus** and **dorsiflexion** may be noted

-**S1** radiculopathy may present w/ pain and paresthesia/numbness along **posterior aspect of leg down to lateral aspect of heel and foot**; **weakness of ankle plantar flexion** may be detected; **ankle jerk reflex** may be absent

-**L4** radiculopathy seen w/ posterolateral disc herniation at L3/4 may present w/ pain and paresthesia/numbness along **anterolateral thigh and below knee to medial aspect of leg and foot**; **weakness of quadriceps** and **knee extension** may be noted

-**L3** radiculopathy, pain and paresthesia may be localized over **anteromedial thigh**

-**L2** distribution presents *over* the **groin**; *both* **L2 and L3** radiculopathies *may* cause **quadriceps weakness**

Relationships with patients

-a psychiatrist **shall NOT gratify his/her own needs by exploiting a patient**; particularly, the impact of one's conduct on the doctor-patient relationship and well-being of the patient

-**sexual activity** w/ current or former patients is **unethical**

-psychiatrist should NOT use the unique position of power afforded by the psychotherapeutic situation to influence patients in any way NOT directly relevant to tx goals

Reliability

-concerns whether or not the findings of an assessment instrument or diagnostic procedure are **reproducible** and can be **replicated** when **instrument is used by different examiners** (*interrater* reliability) or on **different occasions** (*test-retest* reliability)

-effective assessment instrument must be **reliable, valid,** and **free of bias**

Resistance and Defense Mechanisms, psychotherapy

-therapist often point out thoughts and feelings the patient obscures and how they are obscured, defended against, and kept unconscious

-patient's defensive ways of thinking are elucidated in therapy

-therapist identify patterns of defense and resistance and orient the patient to how awareness of these patterns can be used to advance patient's knowledge of him- or herself

-*resistance* refers to all the forces that **oppose painful work of therapy**; serves as protection from experiencing, remembering or reliving, old dangers and fears a/w childhood conflicts and developmental difficulties of his or her life

-many different categories of resistance:

general **fear of any change**;

overly harsh conscience that punishes a patient w/ the continuation of suffering;

insistence on the gratification of childish impulses that forms part of an emotional illness

-ALL people employ **defense mechanisms** to **keep painful feelings and memories *outside* conscious awareness**

-defense mechanisms are specific, discrete maneuvers or ways of thinking that the mind employs to avoid painful emotional material

-character (set of expectable responses from a person in a given setting) is in great part a result of defense mechanisms each person characteristically uses

-**defenses** are our cognitive mechanisms of structuring mental and emotional experience to **keep psychic pain at a minimum** and bring our interpersonal and intrapsychic functioning and relationships *into* some **congruence w/ external reality**

-patient's defense mechanisms are an **important source of resistance** in psychotherapy

Schema

-originally described by **Piaget**

-defined as the **mental representation** of an associated **set of perceptions, ideas,** and/or **actions**

-describes both the mental and physical actions **involved in understanding and knowing**

-categories of knowledge that help us to **interpret and understand the world**

-includes both a **category of knowledge** and the **process of obtaining that knowledge**

-new information is used to modify, add to, or change previously existing schemas as new events occur

Schizophrenia, Bleuler definition

-**Bleuler** coined term "schizophrenia"

-*replaced* dementia precox in the literature

-chose term to express presence of schisms b/w thought, emotion, and behavior in patients w/ the disorder

-stressed that, unlike Kraepelin's concept of dementia precox, schizophrenia need not have a deteriorating course

-often misconstrued by lay people to mean split personality

-split personality (dissociative identity d/o) in DSM-IV-TR differs completely from schizophrenia

Schizophrenia risk, genetic syndromes

-positive association studies have been found for candidate genes implicated in adults

-include **dysbindin** gene, **neuregulin** gene, *DAOA/G30*, *GAD1*, *Prodh2/DGCR6*, and *DISC1*

-youth w/ childhood onset schizophrenia appear to have higher rate of cytogenetic abnormalities than reported in adults w/ schizophrenia; includes **22q11 deletion** syndrome

- **~10-30%** of **22q11.2 deletion** syndrome (**velocardiofacial** or **DiGeorge syndrome**) develop **schizophrenia**-*like* psychotic d/o

Schizophrenia, misdiagnosis in African Americans

-studies demonstrate **overdiagnosis of schizophrenia** and underdiagnosis of affective disorder in **African Americans**

-researchers have found removal of schizoaffective d/o patients from sample strengthen ethnic/racial difference in direction of African American and Latino patients having higher rates of misdiagnosis than white patients

-studies suggest that overdiagnosis of schizophrenia in African Americans is less likely to include schizoaffective d/o

-**cultural differences and clinician biases** complicate relationship b/w psychiatric sxs and diagnoses in African Americans; sxs such as paranoia, which is traditionally a/w schizophrenia may actually reflect depression among African Americans

-research has shown clinicians overdiagnose schizophrenia in African American patients because **mood sxs are *often* overlooked** during admissions to psychiatric hospitals

Serotonin Syndrome

-results from excess serotonergic stimulation; may be seen when transitioning b/w medications or adding medication

-can range in severity from mild to life-threatening

-most common sxs are **delirium**, **rigidity**, **hyperpyrexia**, **confusion**, **flushing**, **diaphoresis**, **tremor**, and **myoclonic jerks** (mental status change; GI sxs; behavioral manifestations; neurological findings; and autonomic abnormalities

-*discontinuation* **of serotonergic medications** is first step, followed by emergency medical tx

-serotonin type 2A (**5-HT$_{2A}$**) receptor *antagonist* **cyproheptadine** can be used if further tx is warranted, beginning w/ oral dose of 12 mg and then administering 2 mg every 2 hours

-tablets may be crushed, mixed in a suspension, and administered via a nasogastric tube; efficacy for this presumed antidote has not been established

Sexual Aversion Disorder
-one of 2 recognized sexual desire disorders:

Hypoactive Sexual Desire Disorder (**more common**)

-characterized by deficiency or absence of sexual fantasies and desire for sexual activity; **more common among women**

Sexual Aversion Disorder

-characterized by **persistent** or **recurrent extreme** *aversion* to, and *avoidance* of, *all* (or almost all) **genital sexual contact w/sexual partner** or by masturbation

-disturbance causes marked distress or interpersonal difficulty

-sexual dysfunction is NOT better accounted for by another Axis I d/o (except another sexual dysfunction)

NOTE:

-minimal spontaneous sexual thinking or minimal desire for sex *ahead* of sexual experiences does *not* necessarily constitute a desire disorder in women, particularly *if* desire is triggered during sexual encounter

-low desire has been reported by 10-15% of women in various countries; in U.S., ~20% of persons have hypoactive sexual desire d/o

Side Effects of SSRIs
-most notably **gastrointestinal problems**, **sexual dysfunction**, and **sleep disturbances**

-considerable differences in SSRI profiles; switch to another SSRI may alleviate or resolve adverse effect

-**sertraline** has a *higher* risk of **diarrhea**, but does NOT usually lead to discontinuation

-**paroxetine** has more **anticholinergic side effects** than other SSRIs; higher affinity for muscarinic receptors

-**weight gain** and **sedating effect** has been found to be *more* **significant w/ paroxetine** than w/ fluoxetine or sertraline, may be d/t **anticholinergic** action

-patient w/ insomnia, may benefit from taking paroxetine at bedtime or switching to less activating SSRI (citalopram or escitalopram)

-excessive activation (significant insomnia) may be warning sign of undiagnosed bipolar d/o; careful screening prior to switching or adding hypnotic

-Insomnia can also be managed by adding a short course of trazodone to drug regimen or by switching patient to mirtazapine or tricyclic antidepressant (TCA)

-**augmentation** w/ either **bupropion** or **mirtazapine** *may* **alleviate sexual side effects**; should be tried prior to switching

Sleep architecture, Elderly
-sleep patterns change over an individual's life span

-adult sleep architecture:

NREM, 75%

Stage 1, 5%

Stage 2, 45%

Stage 3, 12%

Stage 4, 13%

REM, 25%

-sleep architecture remains relatively constant w/ aging

-in elderly; *increased* percentage of time spent in **Stage 1**, *reduction* occurs in *both* **slow-wave sleep** (Stages 3 & 4) secondary to *reduction* in **delta wave amplitude** and **REM** sleep

Smoking rates, young adults
-**young adults 18-24 yrs**, *highest* **rates** of smoking among age groups

-*both* **males and females** in this age group smoked at higher rates than their older counterparts

Social phobia and specific phobia, differential diagnosis
-need to be differentiated from appropriate fear and normal shyness

-DSM-IV-TR aids in the differentiation by requiring that the sxs **impair the patient's ability to function** appropriately

-nonpsychiatric **medical conditions** that can result in development of a phobia *include* use of substances (particularly hallucinogens and sympathomimetics), CNS tumors, and CV dz

-**schizophrenia**; can have phobic sxs as part of their psychoses; patients w/phobia have insight into irrationality of their fears and lack bizarre quality and other psychotic sxs

-**panic d/o**; **agoraphobia**, and **avoidant PD**; patients w/specific phobia or nongeneralized social phobia tend to experience anxiety immediately when presented w/ phobic stimulus; anxiety or panic is limited to identified situation; patients are not abnormally anxious when they are neither confronted w/ phobic stimulus nor caused to anticipate stimulus

-patient w/ agoraphobia is often comforted by presence of another person in anxiety-provoking situation; patient w/ social phobia is made more anxious than before by presence of others

-panic d/o and agoraphobia present w/ breathlessness, dizziness, sense of suffocation, and fear of dying vs. social phobia presentation of blushing, muscle twitching, and anxiety about scrutiny

-*differentiation* **b/w social phobia and avoidant PD can be difficult** and can require extensive interviews and psychiatric hx

Social referencing
-in **second year of life**, child looks to parent and others for **emotional cues** about **how to respond** to novel events

-generally evident by **12 months of age**

Socioeconomic status, stressful life events

-some stressors are so powerful that they evoke significant emotional distress in most o/w mentally healthy people

-majority of stressful life events **do *not* invariably trigger** mental disorders

-more likely to spawn mental disorders in people who are ***vulnerable* biologically**, **socially**, and/or **psychologically**

-groups at *greater* statistical risk include **women**, **young** and **unmarried** people, **African Americans**, and individuals w/ **lower socioeconomic status**

Sodium ion channel gene mutation, periodic paralyses (PP)

-most cases of **hyperkalemic PP** are d/t 2 mutations in *SCN4A*, *T704M*, and *M1592V*

-**mutations in sodium channel**, especially at residues 1448 and 1313, are responsible for **paramyotonia congenita**

-small proportion of hypokalemic periodic paralysis cases are a/w mutations at codons 669 and 672 (HypoPP2); in HypoPP2, sodium channel mutations enhance inactivation to produce net loss of function defect

-**all periodic paralyses** (PPs) are characterized by **episodic weakness; strength is normal b/w attacks**; fixed weakness may develop later in some forms

-most patients w/ primary PP develop sxs before the third decade of life

Hyperkalemic periodic paralyses

-age at onset < 10 yrs

-usually describe sense of heaviness or stiffness in muscles

-weakness starts in thighs and calves, which then spreads to arms and neck

-proximal weakness predominates; distal muscles may become involved after vigorous exercise

-in children, myotonic lid lag (lagging of upper eyelid on downward gaze) may be earliest symptom

-complete paralysis is rare and some residual mobility remains

-respiratory muscle involvement is rare

-attacks last < 4 hrs and in majority of cases, < 1 hr

-sphincters are not involved; any bowel and bladder dysfunction d/t abdominal muscle weakness

-weakness occurs during rest after period of strenuous exercise or during fasting

-may be provoked by potassium, cold, ethanol, or stress

-may be relieved by mild prolonged exercise or carbohydrate intake

Paramyotonia congenita

-autosomal dominant inherited d/o, myotonia worsens w/ activity (paradoxical myotonia) or cold temperatures

-sxs most pronounced in face

-episodic weakness may develop after exercise or cold temperatures and usually lasts a few minutes, but may last as long as days

-potassium loading usually worsens sxs but lowering serum potassium level may precipitates attacks

Stiff-Person syndrome
-characterized by muscle rigidity that waxes and wanes w/ concurrent spasms

-usually *begins* in **axial muscles** and *extends* to **proximal limb muscles**

-**lumbar lordosis** becomes exaggerated *while* **walking**

-severity of the limb muscle involvement may overwhelm axial muscle involvement (stiff limb syndrome)

-EMG shows *no* evidence of distal motor nerve abnormality

-serum *may* be **positive** for anti-glutamic acid decarboxylase (**GAD**) **antibodies**

-pathophysiology of the dz is **autoimmune**

-a/w non-neurologic diseases, including diabetes mellitus and thyroiditis

Stimulant (cocaine and amphetamine) intoxication

-similar sxs w/ **differences in clinical presentation d/t half-lives** of the drugs

-**half-life** for **cocaine, ~40-60 minutes; methamphetamine**, 6-12 hours

-binging common w/both; difference in half-lives allows some methamphetamine abusers to maintain low levels of intoxication for longer periods

-chronic administration of either drug can induce a **paranoid psychotic state**

-some evidence that **methamphetamine-induced psychosis can be long lasting** and *may* **recur in** *absence* **of further drug use**

-individuals may be at **risk of acting violently in response to frightening delusions** common in induced paranoia

-amphetamine use can also result in **delirium** manifested by disorientation, confusion, fear, and anxiety

Stroke, acute treatment with fibrinolytic therapy

-tissue plasminogen activator (**tPA**), **FDA-approved** for *acute* **tx w/in 4 ½ hrs of onset**

-ALL patients w/o contraindications should be offered acute tx w/ tPA

-1/3 of tPA tx'd more likely to have minimal to no deficits at 90 days vs. controls

Indications

-ischemic stroke **w/in 3 hrs of sxs onset**; UNLESS > 80 yrs, ALL patients taking oral anticoagulants regardless of international normalized ratio (INR), baseline National Institutes of Health Stroke Scale (NIHSS) score > 25, hx of stroke and diabetes

-NIHSS > 3

-NO hemorrhage on head CT

-clearly demarcated time of onset

Contraindications

-rapidly resolving deficits

-seizure at onset

-prior stroke or head trauma < 3 mos

-major surgery < 14 days

-prior intracranial hemorrhage

-systolic BP > 185, diastolic BP > 110

-GI or urinary tract hemorrhage < 21 days

-noncompressible arterial puncture < 7 days

-elevated prothrombin time (PT)/partial thromboplastin time (PTT)

-platelets < 100,000, glucose < 50 or > 400

-relative contraindications include NIHSS > 22, CT demonstrating > 1/3 involvement of MCA territory

-do not administer to individuals that awakened w/ stroke sxs unless previously normal on examination w/in previous 3 hrs

Substance dependence, course specifiers

-following Remission specifiers can be applied only after no criteria for Dependence or Abuse have been met for at least 1 month

-specifiers do *not* apply if individual is on agonist therapy or in a controlled environment

-**Early *Full*** Remission. This specifier is used if, for at least 1 month, but for less than 12 months, no criteria for Dependence or Abuse have been met

-**Early *Partial*** Remission. This specifier is used if, for at least 1 month, but less than 12 months, one or more criteria for Dependence or Abuse have been met (but the full criteria for Dependence have *not* been met)

-**Sustained *Full*** Remission. This specifier is used if none of the criteria for Dependence or Abuse have been met at any time during a period of 12 months or longer

-**Sustained *Partial*** Remission. This specifier is used if full criteria for Dependence have not been met for a period of 12 months or longer; however, one or more criteria for Dependence or Abuse have been met

-following specifiers apply if individual is on agonist therapy or in controlled environment:

On **Agonist Therapy**; used if individual is on prescribed agonist medication such as methadone; no criteria for Dependence or Abuse have been met for that class of medication for at least past month (except tolerance to, or withdrawal from, the agonist); also applies to being treated for Dependence using partial agonist or agonist/antagonist

In a **Controlled Environment**; used if individual is in environment where access to alcohol and controlled substances is restricted; no criteria for Dependence or Abuse have been met for at least past month; examples are closely supervised and substance-free jails, therapeutic communities, or locked hospital units

Substance related disorders, violence against others
-most individuals that commit violence have not been dx'd w/ a mental illness

-data clarifying **relationship b/w mental illness and violence** is *limited*

-**most common** psychiatric dx **a/w violence** are **substance related disorders**

-in absence of substance related d/o, individuals w/ major mental illness, such as affective disorders and schizophrenia are **NOT violent**

Substance-Induced Mood Disorder
-must always be considered in differential dx of mood d/o sxs

-consider 3 possibilities:

1) may be taking drugs for **tx of nonpsychiatric medical problems**

2) accidentally or unknowingly, **exposed to neurotoxic chemicals**

3) may have taken substance for **recreational purposes** or be **dependent** on substance

-should **specify substance** involved, time of **onset** (during intoxication or withdrawal), and nature of sxs, **manic or depressed**

-maximum of **1 month b/w use of substance** and **appearance of sxs** is allowed in DSM-IV-TR, timeframe is usually much shorter

-manic and depressive features *can be identical* to those of bipolar I d/o and MDD

-may show more waxing and waning of sxs and fluctuation in patient's level of consciousness

-family hx may indicate likely underlying primary mood disorder but does not rule out possibility of substance-induced mood d/o

-normal mood usually returns shortly after substance has been cleared from body

-occasionally, substance exposure precipitates a longer duration of sxs that may take weeks or months to resolve completely

Suicide risk assessment, legal protection of psychiatrist
-core competency psychiatrists are expected to acquire during residency training

-purpose is to **identify modifiable**, **treatable risk and protective factors** that *inform* patient's **tx and safety management** needs

-*standard of care* **does NOT exist for prediction of suicide**; attempting to predict who will commit suicide creates false-positive and false-negative predictions

-standard of care for suicide risk assessment reveals differences of opinion among competent clinicians, academics, and researchers who testify as experts in suicide cases; clinicians are *expected* **to perform reasonable suicide risk assessments**

-number of suicide risk assessment methods have been proposed; *no* **suicide risk assessment method has been empirically tested for reliability and validity**

-clinicians can create their own systematic suicide risk assessment methodology reflecting their training, clinical experience, and knowledge of evidence-based psychiatric literature

-systematic suicide risk assessment should more than meet standard of care; encourages clinician to gather sufficient information to perform competent assessment

-risk and protective factors are **assessed dimensionally** as **low**, **moderate**, or **high** according to clinical presentation; an overall assessment of level of suicide risk is determined

-assessment of suicide risk and protective factors creates an individualized mosaic of the patient's overall suicide risk

-clinician assesses acute high-risk suicide factors, especially response to tx, over patient's clinical course; protective factors are also monitored

-*acute* is defined as the magnitude and intensity of the symptom, for example, early-morning waking **versus debilitating global insomnia**; a high-risk factor is supported by evidence-based strong a/w suicide

-*no* **form or protocol can encompass ALL possible risk factors**; using standalone risk assessment forms may lead to robotic assessments that fail to capture highly individual risk and protective factors presented by every patient at risk for suicide

-**standardized suicide risk prediction scales do** *not* **identify which patient will attempt or commit suicide**; structured or semistructured suicide scales **may complement but are NOT a substitute for systematic suicide risk assessment**

-**failing to perform a reasonable suicide risk assessment can harm the patient**; suicide risk assessment is an **integral part of psychiatric examination**

-professional organizations have developed practice guidelines for assessment and management of individuals at risk for suicide (American Academy of Child and Adolescent Psychiatry, 2001; American Psychiatric Association, 2003)

Supportive psychotherapy, primary goal

-dyadic tx that uses direct measures to ameliorate sxs and **maintain**, **restore**, or **improve self-esteem**, **ego function**, and adaptive skills (Pinsker 1997; Pinsker et al. 1991; Winston et al. 2004)

-objective is *not* to change patient's personality but to **help patient cope w/ sxs**, **prevent relapse of serious mental illness**, or help a relatively healthy person **deal w/ a crisis or transient problem**

-praise, advice, exhortation, and encouragement, embedded in psychodynamic understanding and used to tx severely impaired patients

Suprascapular lesion/neuropathy

-mixed nerve that provides motor innervation of supraspinatus and infraspinatus muscles and sensory and proprioceptive innervation of posterior aspect of glenohumeral joint, as well as acromioclavicular joint, subacromial bursa, and scapula

-carries afferents from ~ 70% of shoulder joint

-arises from upper trunk of brachial plexus and is composed predominantly of C5-C6 level fibers

-atrophy of supraspinatus and/or infraspinatus muscles may be present on physical exam (depending on site of nerve entrapment)

-relative **weakness of *ipsilateral* shoulder abduction** (function of supraspinatus muscle in addition to deltoid muscle) and/or **weakness of external rotation** (function of infraspinatus muscle in addition to teres minor muscle)

-may report worsening pain w/ cross-body adduction of ipsilateral upper limb

-pressure applied over suprascapular or spinoglenoid notches may elicit pain

-muscle stretch reflexes are unaffected

-rarely, cutaneous appreciation of sensory modalities may be affected in an approximate axillary nerve distribution

Susto, Culture-bound syndrome

-"**fright**," or "**soul loss**;" folk illness prevalent among some **Latinos** in U.S. and people in Mexico, Central America, and South America

-illness **attributed to frightening event** that causes the **soul to leave the body** and results in **unhappiness and sickness**

-also experience significant **strains in key social roles**

-sxs may appear any time; **days to years after fright** is experienced

-believed that death may occur in extreme cases

-typical sxs include appetite disturbances, inadequate or excessive sleep, nightmares, feeling of sadness, lack of motivation, and feelings of low self-worth or dirtiness

-somatic sxs may include muscle aches and pains, headache, stomachache, and diarrhea

-**ritual healings** are focused on **calling the soul back** to the body and **cleansing** the person to **restore bodily and spiritual balance**

-may be *related* to MDD, PTSD, and Somatoform D/O

T

Temperament categories, Thomas and Chess

-began as the New York Longitudinal study in the early 1950s; infant temperament (Thomas, Chess & Birch, 1968) and how well a child fits in at school, w/ friends, and at home

Categories of temperament:

1. activity level

2. regularity of wake/sleep, hunger, bowel movements

3. initial reaction

4. adaptability

5. intensity of emotion

6. mood

7. distractibility

8. persistence and attention span

9. sensitivity (or threshold of responsiveness)

-focused on how temperamental qualities influence adjustment throughout life

-behaviors for each trait on a *continuum*

-tendency toward high or low ends of the scale are a cause for concern

-infants can be categorized into one of **3 groups**: *easy*, *difficult*, and *slow-to-warm-up* (Thomas & Chess 1977)

-*easy* **babies** readily **adapt to new experiences**, generally display positive moods and emotions and also have normal eating and sleeping patterns

-*difficult* **babies** tend to be **very emotional, irritable and fussy, and cry frequently**; irregular eating and sleeping patterns are common

-*slow-to-warm-up* **babies** have a **low activity level and tend to withdraw from new situations and people**; while slow to adapt to new experiences, they generally accept them after repeated exposure

-Chess and colleagues found that these broad patterns are remarkably stable through childhood

-traits tend to be found in children across ALL cultures

Temporal or Giant Cell Arteritis, clinical description/treatment

-should be *considered* in **differential dx of new-onset headache** in **elderly** w/ *elevated* **erythrocyte sedimentation rate**

-dz of cellular immunity; **vasculitic damage** mediated by activated $CD4^+$ T helper cells responding to antigen presented by macrophages; affects internal elastic lamina

-**multinucleated giant cells**, histologic hallmark w/ **temporal artery biopsy**

-superficial temporal artery involved in most patients; predilection for internal elastic lamina, includes aortic arch and branches

-most commonly reported sxs; **headache**; neck, torso, shoulder, and pelvic girdle pain consistent w/ **polymyalgia rheumatica**; fatigue and malaise; **jaw claudication**; fever

-Amaurosis fugax occurs in 10% overall; some degree of permanent **visual loss** occurs in 8%

-**oral corticosteroids** remain mainstay of tx; higher doses of steroids are required to prevent irreversible ischemic ophthalmologic and neurologic complications

-headache and PMR, although most common sxs, are NOT reasons for using high doses of steroids

Thematic Apperception Test

-widely used *projective* process for assessing **patient's self-concept** in **relation to others**

-originally developed by Murray (1943)

-test consists of a set of **30 pictures** depicting one or more individuals; patient is asked to **make up a story based on each picture**

-stories generated are scored for individual's needs as reflected in *feelings and impulses* **attributed to major character in each story** and *interactions* **w/ the environment** leading to a resolution

-stories generated are examined for patient's self-other concepts as revealed in interaction and outcome of story line

Thought Content
-description should include:

Mention of **important themes**

Presence or absence of **delusional or obsessional thinking** and **suicidal or homicidal thoughts**

-*delusional* thinking includes **fixed false beliefs** that are **persecutory**, **erotomanic**, **grandiose**, **somatic**, or **jealous** in content

Patients *believe* their **fixed false beliefs** *are reality*

Thought disorders (schizophrenia or schizoaffective d/o) are **most likely cause of bizarre** delusions **over long period of time**

-**alcohol or drug intoxication may cause** *acute* **changes** in thought content, including paranoid ideation or even delusional thinking

-*obsessions* are defined as **recurrent, persistent thoughts that intrude involuntarily** into a person's thinking; **senseless** and are *not* **based in reality**

-obsessions are common w/ OCD, also occur in eating d/o or impulse control d/o; intrusive thoughts are recognized by individual as *not* normal, as opposed to believing them to be reality, distinguishes obsessions from delusions

Thyroid dysfunction and depression
-*undetected* thyroid dysfunction found in 5-10% of depressed patients

-20-30% have blunted TSH response w/ TRH challenge, *suggestive* of hyperthyroidism but *rare* in depressed patients; thought to be from downregulation at pituitary level

Tics and Attention-Deficit Hyperactivity Disorder treatment with stimulants

-recent studies indicate **chronic** tic disorders occur in **1-3% of school children** and ~1/4 of children requiring **special education** services

-**21-90%** of children **w/ Tourette's Syndrome** have **comorbid ADHD**

-frequency of **tic worsening** (20%) was **no higher** for subjects **treated w/ methylphenidate** than for those receiving placebo (22%) or clonidine alone (26%)

-indicates **tic accentuation** may **NOT** be a **direct pharmacologic effect** of medication

Tobacco dependence, CYP2A6 gene inactive alleles

-**CYP2A6** enzyme mediates **> 90% of conversion of nicotine to cotinine, major route of elimination of nicotine**

-CYP2A6 activity is important **indicator of *susceptibility* to tobacco dependence**

-studies have found that slowest CYP2A6 activity may be protective for being a current adult smoker, suggesting possible tobacco dependence protective effect of the slow CYP2A6-mediated nicotine metabolism; some *conflicting* study results

-slow rate of nicotine conversion into cotinine results in prolonged presence of higher nicotine concentrations in blood, **increased level of cotinine per unit drug ingested**; increases exposure of nicotinic acetylcholine receptors in brain to nicotine

Toddler (18 mos-3 yrs), development of symbolic representation and language

-ability to **form symbols** emerges; toddlers' *cannot* distinguish b/w symbol and what it symbolizes, may attribute **lifelike qualities to inanimate objects, *animism***

-by 2 years, toddlers' ability to form symbolic conceptions and learn words enables them ability to **understand concepts expressed in verbal language**

Topographical Model of the Mind

-described by **Freud**, *The Interpretation of Dreams* (1900); divided mind into **3 regions**: *conscious* system, *preconscious* system, and *unconscious* system

Conscious

-part of mind in which **perceptions coming from *outside* world or from *w/in* the body or mind** are **brought *into* awareness**; content can be communicated only by means of language or behavior

-uses a form of neutralized psychic energy, ***attention cathexis***, in which individuals are aware of particular idea or feeling as a result of investing a discrete amount of psychic energy in the idea or feeling

Preconscious

-composed of mental events, processes, and contents that can be **brought *into* conscious awareness** by **act of focusing attention**

-most persons can recall information or images that they are NOT consciously aware of but can bring the information or image to mind by deliberately focusing attention on the memory

-interfaces w/ both unconscious and conscious regions of the mind; to reach conscious awareness, contents of unconscious must become linked w/ words to become preconscious

-also serves to maintain repressive barrier and censor unacceptable wishes and desires

Unconscious

-dynamic system; mental contents and processes are **kept from conscious awareness** through force of **censorship or repression**; closely related to instinctual drives

-was thought to contain primarily mental representations and derivatives of sexual instinct

-content of unconscious is limited to wishes seeking fulfillment; provide motivation for dream and neurotic symptom formation; view is now considered reductionist

-characterized by ***primary process* thinking**, aimed at facilitating wish fulfillment and instinctual discharge; governed by pleasure principle and disregards logical connections; has no concept of time, represents wishes as fulfillments, permits contradictions to exist simultaneously, and denies existence of negatives

-memories in unconscious have been divorced from connection w/ verbal symbols

-contents of unconscious can become conscious only by passing through preconscious when censors are overpowered

Limitations

-2 main deficiencies realized by Freud; conflict b/w defense mechanisms not being accessible to consciousness and incompatibility b/w repression and preconscious

-despite limitations of topographical theory, concepts from theory continue to be useful; primary and secondary thought processes; fundamental importance of wish fulfillment; existence of dynamic unconscious; tendency toward regression under frustrating conditions

Tourette syndrome, treatment of motor and vocal tics

-essential to assess impact of tic disorder on person's quality of life and overall psychological adjustment

-persistent tics, tx decisions are often based on severity of persistent tics, psychiatric comorbidity, and degree of interference w/work or social interaction

-tx planning requires thorough understanding of tic disorder's natural course; relationship to person's developmental, psychosocial, and academic needs and stressors; severity of abnormal movements and vocalizations; disruptive sxs (e.g., coprolalia, copropraxia); psychiatric comorbidity; and risk–benefit ratio of available tx

-waxing and waning course of tic disorders can make it difficult to assess effectiveness of tx

-many clinicians use one of the **alpha$_2$-noradrenergic agents** (**guanfacine, clonidine**) as their **first choice**, for milder tics, safer for chronic use and have fewer SE than antipsychotics

-usual daily dose of guanfacine is 1-3 mg in 2 to 3 divided doses; usual dose of clonidine is 0.1-0.3 mg in 3 to 4 divided doses; *may* **take several weeks to see full effect**

-principal side effect is **dose-related sedation**; **hypotension** is usually not a problem w/careful dosing

-**haloperidol** and **pimozide** studied *more* than any other agents; **TD** are **rare in children on *low* doses of antipsychotics** for relatively *brief* periods of time

-risperidone, olanzapine, and ziprasidone have been shown to be useful for tics in controlled studies; share troublesome short-term side effects of older typical antipsychotics; ECG monitoring for QTc prolongation is essential w/pimozide and ziprasidone, and caution is necessary regarding coadministration of medications (such as macrolide antibiotics and some SSRIs that may interfere w/cytochrome metabolism, can result in fatal arrhythmias

-80% of Tourette's d/o patients will benefit from haloperidol or pimozide, w/mean reduction of sxs of 65%; haloperidol, fluphenazine, and pimozide produce significant adverse effects, especially sedation or cognitive blunting, w/ as many as 50% of patients developing side effects

-clonazepam has been used as adjunctive tx for tics

Transference, Psychodynamic therapy

-displacement of feelings and thoughts a/w a figure in **patient's past** *onto* **the therapist**

-often **unconscious** initially; patient may be bewildered by behavior toward the therapist because it does not make sense

-*hallmark* of **psychodynamic** or psychoanalytic psychotherapy

Tricyclic and tetracyclic antidepressants, blood levels

-ECG can assess for **conduction delays** *before* starting a regimen of cyclic drugs, which *may* lead to **heart block at therapeutic levels**

-some clinicians recommend annual ECG in patients receiving prolonged cyclic drug therapy

-at therapeutic levels, these drugs suppress arrhythmias through quinidine-like effect

-blood levels should be determined *routinely* when using **imipramine, desipramine,** or **nortriptyline** in tx of depressive d/o

-can be useful in patient w/poor response at normal dosage range

-blood level determinations should also include measurement of active metabolites (e.g., imipramine is converted to desipramine, amitriptyline [Elavil] to nortriptyline)

Imipramine

-percentage of favorable responses correlates w/ plasma levels in linear manner b/w **200-250 ng/mL**; levels > 250 ng/mL yield no greater benefit, adverse effects increase

Nortriptyline

-therapeutic window b/w **50-150 ng/mL**; response rate decreases at levels > 150 ng/mL

Desipramine

-levels > **125 ng/mL** correlate w/higher percentage of favorable responses

Amitriptyline

-*conflicting* results w/ regard to blood levels; range from **75-175 ng/mL**

Procedure for **Determining Blood Concentrations**

-should be drawn **10-14 hrs after last dose**, *usually* in AM after bedtime dose

-must have received **stable daily dose for *at least* 5 days** for test to be valid

-patients who metabolize cyclic drugs unusually poorly may have levels as high as 2,000 ng/mL while taking normal dosages and before showing a favorable clinical response; must be monitored closely for cardiac adverse effects

-levels > **1,000 ng/mL** are generally *at risk* **for cardiotoxicity**

Trigeminal neuralgia or Tic Douloureux, clinical presentation
-presents characteristically as **severe**, paroxysmal, and **lancinating unilateral facial pain**

-triggered by chewing or similar activities or touching affected areas on face

-can **localize pain precisely**; pain not confined exclusively to one of 3 divisions of nerve

-commonly runs along line dividing either mandibular and maxillary nerves or mandibular and ophthalmic portions of trigeminal nerve

-**60%** complain of lancinating pain shooting from **corner of mouth to angle of jaw**

-**30%** experience jolts of pain from **upper lip or canine teeth to eye and eyebrow**, sparing orbit itself; distribution falls b/w division of first and second portions of trigeminal nerve

-when unilateral, affects right side of face 5 times more frequently than left

-typically starts w/ sensation of electrical shocks in affected area, then quickly escalates into excruciating discomfort felt deep in the face in < 20 seconds; pain begins to fade w/in seconds and gives way to burning ache lasting seconds to minutes

-characteristic grimace during attacks; "**tic douloureux**"

-number of attacks may vary from < 1 per day to 12 or more per hour, up to hundreds per day

-affected individuals avoid rubbing the face or shaving trigger area; may hold face still while talking to avoid precipitating attack

-**chewing**, **talking**, **smiling**, **wind** blowing on cheek, or **drinking cold or hot fluids** *may* **initiate pain**

-may remit for months or years after initial attack

-may find immediate relief w/ **carbamazepine**; **gabapentin** has been more widely used recently d/t reduced side effects although considered less effective than carbamazepine

-chronically, *may require* a second or third drug to control episodes and possibly surgical intervention

U

Ulnar nerve lesion

-injury from trauma or compression

-may occur where it passes through ulnar groove of elbow or more distally in cubital tunnel

-may occur when individual rest arm's weight on their elbows

-develop **atrophy**, particularly **hypothenar** eminence, and **weakness** of **hand muscles**, "claw hand"

-**fourth and fifth fingers** *flexed* and *abducted*

-loss of sensation in fourth and fifth fingers and medial surface of the hand

-once common among watchmakers and dubbed, "watchmaker's palsy"

V

Validity, assessment instruments
-concerns whether a test **measures what it is *supposed* to measure**

-does the assessment instrument *identify* **cases** it is **designed to identify**

external validity, does the study population *represent* the population to be treated

internal validity, can observed changes or differences in the dependent variable confidently be attributed to the independent variable (experimental drug, etc.)

criterion validity, results from one test instrument are compared w/ results of another test whose validity has already been established

face validity, test makes sense to the investigator using it

content validity, test covers specific types of information that can be interpreted or scored at a later date

concurrent validity, results correspond to results of another test w/ same variable

construct validity, test instrument is in fact measuring what it was designed to measure

-properties of validity and reliability are extremely important in psychiatric epidemiology; especially if attempting to identify a specific disorder or syndrome

Valproate, dosage and clinical guidelines
-*prior* to initiating; standard **chemistry** screen w/ **LFTs, CBC, platelet count,** and **pregnancy test**

-during tx; LFTs at 1 month, then every 6-24 months if no abnormalities; CBC, platelet count at 1 month, then every 6-24 months if no abnormalities

-abnormal LFTs; mild transaminase elevation (< 3x normal), monitoring every 1-2 weeks, if stable and patient is responding to valproate, results are monitored monthly to every 3 months

-*marked* **LFT elevation (> 3x normal); dosage reduction** *or* **discontinue** valproate; then **increase dose or rechallenge if LFTs** *normalize* **and if patient is valproate responder**

-frequent monitoring may not predict serious organ toxicity; requires prompt evaluation of any illnesses, asymptomatic elevation of **LFTs up to 3x upper limit of normal are common** and **do NOT require any change in dose**

-tx of **acute mania**; **oral loading w/ 20-30 mg/kg a day** can be used to accelerate control of sxs, usually well tolerated but can cause excessive sedation and tremor in elderly

-in absence of acute mania; best to initiate gradually to minimize common adverse effects of nausea, vomiting, and sedation

-dose on **first day** *should* be **250 mg administered w/ meal**; can be increased to 250 mg orally 3 times daily over 3-6 days

-plasma concentrations can be **assessed in AM** *before* **first daily dose**

-therapeutic plasma concentrations for control of seizures, 50-150 µg/mL, concentrations **up to 200 µg/mL usually well tolerated**

-most controlled studies used 50-125 µg/mL; *most* attain therapeutic plasma concentrations at **1,200-1,500 mg/day in divided doses**

-full daily dose can be taken **all at once before sleep** *after* sxs are controlled

Valproate, weight gain

-weight gain is a **common side effect** of valproate tx; **most common reason** patients **discontinue** valproate

-does **NOT** appear to be **dose dependent**

-reported significant weight gain w/ associated hyperinsulinemia in ~50% of a cohort of women taking valproate

-diet and exercise should be recommended early in tx

Variable-ratio schedule

-**operant conditioning** reinforcement schedule in which a reward is given after a **varying number of responses** have been emitted (used in slot machines).

Vascular dementia

-often called multi-infarct dementia

-sometimes further classified as cortical or subcortical dementia

-vascular dz produces either focal or diffuse effects on the brain and causes cognitive decline

-focal CV dz occurs secondary to thrombotic or embolic vascular occlusions

-common areas a/w cognitive decline are the white matter of cerebral hemispheres and the deep gray nuclei, especially striatum and thalamus

-HTN is major cause of diffuse dz, and in many patients, both focal and diffuse dz are observed together

-3 most common mechanisms of vascular dementia are multiple cortical infarcts; strategic single infarct; and small vessel dz

-risk factors include stroke and preexisting cognitive impairment, from Alzheimer's dz

-depression considered another risk factor (more common in vascular dementia)

-typically accompanied by **focal neurologic deficits**, which *differentiates* it **from Alzheimer's dz**; hemiparesis, dysarthria, clumsiness, and gait impairment (place most cases in subcortical category) basal ganglia involvement

-neurologic function often deteriorates in a "stepwise" pattern

-sometimes signs of frontal lobe injury; apathy, emotional instability, impaired executive function, incontinence, and pseudobulbar palsy

Vertebral artery dissection, chiropractic adjustment

-**rare** but potentially disabling; exact incidence is still unknown

-caused by **traumatic** or **spontaneous arterial injury** occurring during or shortly after cervical manipulation

-**vertigo and disequilibrium** are usual presenting sxs, may show **fluctuating course** and misdiagnosed as peripheral vertigo; can result from inner ear or vestibular nerve dysfunction, vertebrobasilar insufficiency, lethal cerebellar infarction or hemorrhage

-**most frequently** reported complication is **posterior circulation stroke** related to **vertebral artery dissection**

Vitamin B12 deficiency; dementia, ataxia, dysesthesia

-neurological signs/sxs may be the earliest, if not only manifestations of deficiency

-often considered **reversible** form of dementia if detected and treated early

-sensory disturbance, including **dysesthesia** or paresthesias, are earliest neurological manifestation

-presence of subacute combined degeneration of spinal cord often present; **weakness**, **areflexia**, *loss* **of position and vibration sense in** *lower* **extremities, bilateral Babinski signs**

-may be a/w **macrocytic** anemia; *elevated* **homocysteine** and **methylmalonic acid** levels

W

Wisconsin Card Sorting Test

-test of **concept formation** and **cognitive flexibility**, and **reasoning**

-subjects **match cards** *according to feedback* **about the** *correctness* of their sorts

-a key feature is that *after* **10 correct sorts**, the *correct* **sorting principle changes** *w/o warning*, and subjects must change their sorting strategy accordingly

-test places a strong emphasis on **cognitive flexibility** and highlights perseverative error because of the lack of warning about the change

Wraparound Services

-helpful when children and families have **significant emotional and behavioral difficulties** and have **experienced tx failures**; goal is to **prevent hospitalizations** or *need* for **residential placement**

-may be involved in foster care, child protective services, juvenile justice, residential tx facilities, and special education

- ~200,000 children in U.S. are served by wraparound services

-consensus group of experts in 1998 came to define key elements of wraparound services; many aspects involve developing a particular perspective and attitude, rather than specifying well-defined components of care

-3 key characteristics of wraparound

1) strength-based orientation

2) value placed on cultural competence

3) integration of family as active participant in building tx plan

-RCTs have found benefits to wraparound services; mixed results include The Fort Bragg Study, although the *tx as usual* was more intensive than many communities

Writ of habeas corpus

-applies to individuals *involuntarily* hospitalized

-if there is a question as to whether the individual has been illegally deprived of liberty to ask for a legal proceeding, **the court** decides if the individual has been **hospitalized** *w/o due process* **of law**

Bibliography

Agency for Healthcare Research and Quality. *Newer class of antidepressants similar in effectiveness, but side effects differ*. January 24, 2007. Available at: http://www.ahrq.gov/news/press/pr2007/antideppr.htm. Accessed July 15, 2010.

American Medical Association publication, *Physician's Guide to Counseling and Assessing Older Drivers*. http://www.ama-assn.org/ama/pub/category/10791.html. Accessed July 30, 2010.

American Psychiatric Association. *Diagnostic and Statistical Manual of Mental Disorders: DSM-IV-TR*. 4th ed. Washington: American Psychiatric Association; 2000.

American Psychiatric Association. *Practice guideline for the treatment of patients with obsessive-compulsive disorder*. Arlington, VA: American Psychiatric Association; 2007. Available online at http://www.psychiatryonline.com.

American Psychiatric Association. *Psychiatric Services in Jails and Prisons: A Task Force Report of the American Psychiatric Association*, 2nd Edition. Washington, DC, American Psychiatric Association; 2000.

American Psychiatric Association. *The Principles of Medical Ethics with Annotations Especially Applicable to Psychiatry*. Washington, DC: American Psychiatric Association; 2001.

Anderson HS. Alzheimer disease. eMedicine. http://emedicine.medscape.com/article/1134817-overview. Accessed August 1, 2010.

APA Work Group on Alzheimer's Disease and other Dementias. *American Psychiatric Association practice guideline for the treatment of patients with Alzheimer's disease and other dementias*. Second edition. *Am J Psychiatry*. 2007 Dec;164(12 Suppl):5-56.

Ayd FJ Jr: A survey of drug-induced extrapyramidal reactions. *JAMA* 1961;175:1054-1060.

Baldessarini RJ, Tondo L, Davis P, et al. Decreased risk of suicides and attempts during long-term lithium treatment: a meta-analytic review. *Bipolar Disord* 2006;8:625-639.

Baldisseri MR. Impaired healthcare professional. *Crit Care Med* 2007;35[Suppl.]:S106-S116.

Barnes TRE, Spence SA. Movement disorders associated with antipsychotic drugs: clinical and biological implications, in *Psychopharmacology of Schizophrenia*. Edited by Reverly MA, Deakin JFW. New York, Oxford University Press; 2000:178-210.

Bateman DN, Darling WM, Boys R, Rawlins MD. Extrapyramidal reactions to metoclopramide and prochlorperazine. *QJM* 1989;71:307-11.

Borowitz S. Encopresis. eMedicine. http://emedicine.medscape.com/article/928795-treatment. Accessed August 1, 2010.

Bostwick JM, Hecksel KA, Stevens SR, et al: Frequency of new-onset pathological gambling or hypersexuality after drug treatment of idiopathic Parkinson's disease. *Mayo Clinic Proceedings* 2009; 84:310-316.

Bozorg AM. Restless leg syndrome. eMedicine. http://emedicine.medscape.com/article/1188327-treatment. Accessed July 23, 2010.

Brown J, O' Brien PM, Marjoribanks J, Wyatt K. Selective serotonin reuptake inhibitors for premenstrual syndrome. *Cochrane Database Syst Rev.* Apr 15 2009;CD001396.

Busch KA, Fawcett J, Jacobs DG. Clinical correlates of inpatient suicide. *J Clin Psychiatry* 2003;64:14-19.

Carbamazepine Oral. Monograph – Carbamazepine, drug interactions. Medscape. Accessed at: http://www.medscape.com/druginfo/monograph?cid=med&drugid=1493&drugname=Carbamazepine+Oral &monotype=monograph&secid=5

Chen WL et al. Vertebral artery dissection and cerebellar infarction following chiropractic manipulation. *Emerg Med J.* 2006 January; 23(1):e1.

Child Welfare Information Gateway. Grounds for Involuntary Termination of Parental Rights: Summary of State Laws. U.S. Department of Health and Human Services, June 2007. http://www.childwelfare.gov/systemwide/laws_policies/statutes/groundtermin.cfm. Accessed August 1, 2010.

Chuang DT, Shih VE. Maple syrup urine disease (branched-chain ketoaciduria). In: Scriver CR, Beaudet AL, Sly WS, Valle D (eds) *The Metabolic and Molecular Bases of Inherited Disease.* McGraw-Hill, New York; 2001:1971-2006.

Cipriani A, Pretty H, Hawton K, et al. Lithium in the prevention of suicidal behavior and all-cause mortality in patients with mood disorders: a systematic review of randomized trials. *Am J Psychiatry* 2005;162:1805-1819.

Clarke R et al. Vital Trial Collaborative Group. Effect of vitamins and aspirin on markers of platelet activation, oxidative stress and homocysteine in people at high risk of dementia. *J Intern Med.* 2003;254(1):67-75.

Conrad ME. Pernicious anemia. eMedicine. http://emedicine.medscape.com/article/204930-overview. Accessed August 1, 2010.

Dangond F. Multiple Sclerosis. eMedicine. http://emedicine.medscape.com/article/1146199-overview. Accessed August 21, 2010.

Daviss WB, Bentivoglio P, Racusin R, Brown KM, Bostic JQ, Wiley L. Bupropion sustained release in adolescents with comorbid attention-deficit/hyperactivity disorder and depression. *J Am Acad Child Adolesc Psychiatry*. 2001;40;307-314.

Deisenhammer EA, Huber M, Kemmler G, et al. Psychiatric hospitalizations during the last 12 months before suicide. *Gen Hosp Psychiatry* 2007;29:63-65.

Devine ME, Rands G. Does aspirin affect outcome in vascular dementia? A retrospective case notes analysis. *Int J Geriatr Psychiatry*. 2003;18(5):425-31.

Dieperink E, Ho SB, Tetrick L, et al. Suicidal ideation during interferon-alpha2b and ribavirin treatment of patients with chronic hepatitis C. *Gen Hosp Psychiatry* 2004;26:237-240.

Dollarhide AW, Loh C, Leckband SG, et al. Psychiatric comorbidity does not predict interferon treatment completion rates in hepatitis C-seropositive veterans. *J Clin Gastroenterol* 2007; 41:322-328.

Dording CM, Mischoulon D, Peterson TJ, et al. The pharmacologic management of selective serotonin reuptake inhibitor-induced side effects: a survey of psychiatrists. *Ann Clin Psychiatr*. 2002;14:143-147.

Driver-Dunckley E, Samanta J, Stacy M. Pathological gambling associated with dopamine agonist therapy in Parkinson's disease. *Neurology* 2003;61:422-423.

Duddy ME, Baker MR. Stiff person syndrome. *Front Neurol Neurosci*. 2009;26:147-65.

Dulcan M. *Dulcan's Textbook of Child and Adolescent Psychiatry*. Washington: American Psychiatric Publishing; 2010.

Edwards KR, Hershey L, Wray L, et al. Efficacy and safety of galantamine in patients with dementia with Lewy bodies: a 12-week interim analysis. *Dement Geriatr Cogn Disord* 2004;17 (suppl 1):40-48.

El-Mallakh RS. Complications of concurrent lithium and electroconvulsive therapy: a review of clinical material and theoretical considerations. *Biol Psychiatry* 1988;23:595-601.

Espay AJ. Hydrocephalus. eMedicine. http://emedicine.medscape.com/article/1135286-overview. Accessed July 26, 2010.

Farber NB et al. Serotonergic Agents That Activate $5HT_{2A}$ Receptors Prevent NMDA Antagonist Neurotoxicity. *Neuropsychopharmacology* 1998;18:57-62.

Fawcett J. Suicide risk factors in depressive disorders and panic disorder. *J Clin Psychiatry* 1992;53 (suppl):9-13.

Fawcett J, Scheftner WA, Fogg L, et al. Time-related predictors of suicide in major affective disorders. *Am J Psychiatry* 1991;147:1189-1194.

Filippini G et al. Corticosteroids or ACTH for acute exacerbations in multiple sclerosis. *Cochrane Database Syst Rev* 2010 Issue 7; http://www2.cochrane.org/reviews/en/ab001331.html. Accessed July 27, 2010.

Fokunang et al. Evaluation of hepatotoxicity and nephrotoxicity in HIV patients on highly active anti-retroviral therapy. *Journal of AIDS and HIV Research* March 2010;2(3):48-57. Available online http://www.academicjournals.org/jahr

Fried MW. Side effects of therapy of hepatitis C and their management. *Hepatology* 2002; 36:S237-S244.

Gabbard GO. *Long-Term Psychodynamic Psychotherapy: A Basic Text*, Second Edition. Washington: American Psychiatric Publishing; 2010.

Gabbard GO. *Psychodynamic Psychiatry in Clinical Practice*, 4th Edition. Washington, DC, American Psychiatric Publishing; 2005.

Gabbard GO. *Textbook of Psychotherapeutic Treatments*. Washington: American Psychiatric Publishing; 2009.

Gabbard GO. *The American Psychiatric Publishing Gabbard's Treatments of Psychiatric Disorders*, 4th Edition. Washington: American Psychiatric Publishing; 2007.

Galanter M, Kleber HD. *The American Psychiatric Press Textbook of Substance Abuse Treatment*, 4th ed. Washington, D.C.: American Psychiatric Press; 2008.

Glauser T, Ben Menachem E, Bourgeois B, et al. ILAE treatment guidelines: evidence-based analysis of antiepileptic drug efficacy and effectiveness as initial monotherapy for epileptic seizures and syndromes. *Epilepsia* 2006;47:1094-1120.

Goldfrank LR, Lewin NA, Flomenbaum NE, et al. Antidepressants: tricyclics, tetracyclics, monoamine oxidase inhibitors, and others, in *Goldfrank's Toxicologic Emergencies*, 3rd Edition. Edited by Goldfrank LR, Flomenbaum ME, Lewis NA, et al. Norwalk, CT, Appleton-Century-Crofts, 1986;351-363.

Goodwin DW et al. Alcoholic "blackouts": a review and clinical study of 100 alcoholics. *Am J Psychiatry* 1969;126:191-198.

Goodwin RD, Pine DS. Respiratory disease and panic attacks among adults in the United States. *Chest* 2002;122:645-650.

Grant D, Berg E. A behavioral analysis of the degree of reinforcement and ease of shifting to new responses in a Weigl-type card sorting problem. *J Exp Psychol* 1948;38:404-411.

Griffiths RR, Juliano LM, Chausmer AL. Caffeine pharmacology and clinical effects. In: Graham AW, Schultz TK, Mayo-Smith MF, Ries RK, Wilford BB (eds.). *Principles of Addiction Medicine*, 3rd ed. Chevy Chase, MD: American Society of Addiction; 2003:193-224.

Guzzetta F, Tondo L, Centorrino F, et al. Lithium treatment reduces suicide risk in recurrent major depressive disorder. *J Clin Psychiatry* 2007;68:380-383.

Hales RE, Yudofsky SC. *The American Psychiatric Publishing Textbook of Clinical Psychiatry*. 5th ed. Washington: American Psychiatric Publishing; 2008.

Hayden EP, Klein DN. Predicting the outcome of dysthymic disorder at 5-year follow-up: The impact of familial psychopathology, early adversity, personality, comorbidity, and chronic stress. *Am J Psychiatry*. 2001;158:1864-1870.

Hathaway SR, McKinley JC. *Minnesota Multiphasic Personality Inventory—2*. Minneapolis, University of Minnesota Press; 1989.

Hathaway SR, McKinley JC. *Minnesota Multiphasic Personality Inventory Manual*, Revised Edition. New York, Psychological Corporation; 1967.

Htay TT et al. Premenstrual dysphoric disorder. eMedicine. http://emedicine.medscape.com/article/293257-treatment. Accessed August 1, 2010.

Isometsa ET, Henriksson MM, Heikkinen ME, et al. Suicide among subjects with personality disorders. *Am J Psychiatry*. 1996;153(5):667-673.

Jauch EC, Kissela B. Acute stroke management. eMedicine. http://emedicine.medscape.com/article/1159752-treatment. Accessed August 20, 2010.

Jennison KM, Johnson KA. Drinking-induced blackouts among young adults: results from a national longitudinal study. *Int J Addict*. 1994;29:23-51.

Kagan J, Snidman N, McManis M, et al. Temperamental contributions to the affect family of anxiety. *Psychiatr Clin North Am* 2001;24:677-88.

Kaplan BJ, Sadock VA. *Kaplan and Sadock's Synopsis of Psychiatry*. 10th ed. Philadelphia: Lippincott Williams & Wilkins; 2007.

Kaufman DM. *Clinical Neurology for Psychiatrists*. 6th ed. Philadelphia: WB Saunders; 2007.

Kay J, Tasman A, Lieberman JA. *Psychiatry: Behavioral Science and Clinical Essentials*. Philadelphia: WB Saunders; 1999:204.

Kaye V, Brandstater ME. Transcutaneous Electrical Nerve Stimulation. eMedicine. http://emedicine.medscape.com/article/325107-overview. Accessed August 19, 2010.

Keller MB et al. Double Depression: Two-year follow-up. *Am J Psychiatry*. 1983;140:689-694.

Keller MB et al. Results of the DSM-IV Mood Disorders Field Trial. *Am J Psychiatry*. 1995;152:843-849.

Kessler RC, Coccaro EF, Fava M, Jaeger S, Jin R, Walters E. The prevalence and correlates of DSM-IV intermittent explosive disorder in the National Comorbidity Survey Replication. *Arch Gen Psychiatry* 2006;63(6):669-78.

Kessler RC, Berglund PA, Demler O, Jin R, Walters EE. Lifetime prevalence and age-of-onset distributions of DSM-IV disorders in the National Comorbidity Survey Replication (NCS-R). *Arch Gen Psychiatry*. 2005;62(6):593-602.

Kirshner HS, Jacobs DH. Aphasia. eMedicine. http://emedicine.medscape.com/article/1135944-overview. Accessed July 28, 2010.

Klein DN et al. Ten-year prospective follow-up study of the naturalistic course of dysthymic disorder and double depression. *Am J Psychiatry*. 2006;163:872-880.

Kohut H. *The analysis of the self*. New York: International Universities Press; 1971.

Kovacs M et al. First-episode major depressive and dysthymic disorder in childhood: Clinical and sociodemographic factors in recovery. *Journal of the American Academy of Child and Adolescent Psychiatry*. 1997;36:777-784.

Kübler-Ross E. On Death and Dying. New York: Macmillan; 1969.

Kumar N. Nutritional neuropathies. *Neurol Clin*. 2007;25:209-255.

Lantz PM. Smoking on the rise among young adults: implications for research and policy. Tob Control 2003;12(Suppl 1);i60--i70.

Louis ED, Klatka LA, Liu Y, et al. Comparison of extrapyramidal features in 31 pathologically confirmed cases of diffuse Lewy body disease and 34 pathologically confirmed cases of Parkinson's disease. *Neurology* 1997;48:376-380.

Lovell K, Cox D, Haddock G, Jones C, Raines D, Garvey R, Roberts C, Hadley S. Telephone administered cognitive behaviour therapy for treatment of obsessive compulsive disorder: randomised controlled non-inferiority trial. *BMJ*. 2006;333:883.

Mack A, Franklin JE Jr, Frances RJL. Substance use disorders, in *American Psychiatric Publishing Textbook of Clinical Psychiatry*, 4th Edition. Edited by Hales RE, Yudofsky SC. Washington, DC, American Psychiatric Publishing, 2003; 309-378.

Marangell LB, Martinez JM. *Concise Guide to Psychopharmacology*, 2nd Edition. Arlington, VA, American Psychiatric Publishing; 2006:146-147.

Mayo-Smith MF, Beecher LH, Fischer TL, et al: Management of alcohol withdrawal delirium: an evidence-based practice guideline. *Arch Intern Med* 2004;164:1405-1412.

McKeith I, Mintzer J, Aarsland D, et al. Dementia with Lewy bodies. *Lancet Neurol* 2004;3:19-28.

McKeith IG, Ballard CG, Harrison RW. Neuroleptic sensitivity to risperidone in Lewy body dementia. *Lancet* 1995;346:699.Mersy DJ. Recognition of Alcohol and Substance Abuse. *Am Fam Physician* 2003;67(7):1529-1532.

McLeod JD, Kessler RC. Socioeconomic status differences in vulnerability to undesirable life events. *Journal of Health and Social Behavior* 1990;(31):162-172.

Meltzer HY, Okayli G. Reduction of suicidality during clozapine treatment of neuroleptic-resistant schizophrenia: impact on risk-benefit assessment. *Am J Psychiatry* 1995;152:183-190.

Milberger S, Biederman J, Faraone SV, Murphy J, Tsuang MT. Attention deficit hyperactivity disorder and comorbid disorders: issues of overlapping symptoms. *Am J Psychiatry*. 1995;152:1793-1799.

Miller WR, Rollnick S. *Motivational Interviewing: Preparing People for Change*, 2nd ed. Guilford Press; 2002.

Miranda J, Green BL. The need for mental health services research focusing on poor young women. *Journal of Mental Health Policy and Economics* 1999;(2):73-89.Meltzer HY. Suicidality in schizophrenia: a review of the evidence for risk factors and treatment options. *Curr Psychiatry Rep* 2002;4:279-283.

Mohammad J. Lithium and Psoriasis: What Primary Care and Family Physicians Should Know. *Prim Care Companion J Clin Psychiatry*. 2008;10(6):435-439.

Monnell K, Zachariah SB. Bell palsy. eMedicine. http://emedicine.medscape.com/article/1146903-overview. Accessed August 20, 2010.

Murdoch D, Pihl RO, Ross D. Alcohol and crimes of violence: Present issues. *International Journal of Addictions* 1990;25:1065-1081.

Myrick H, Anton R: Recent advances in the pharmacotherapy of alcoholism. *Curr Psychiatry Rep* 2004;6:332-338.

National Commission on Correctional Health Care. *Correctional Mental Health Care: Standards and Guidelines for Delivering Services*. Chicago, National Commission on Correctional Health Care, 1999.

National Institute of Neurological Disorders and Stroke. *National Institutes of Health. Tremor Fact Sheet, NINDS*. NIH Publication No. 06-4734; Publication date June 2006. Accessed at http://www.ninds.nih.gov/disorders/tremor/detail_tremor.htm

Neighbors HW, Trierweler SJ, Mundav C, et al. Psychiatric diagnosis of African Americans: diagnostic divergence in clinician-structured and semistructured interviewing conditions. *J Natl Med Assoc*. 1999;91:601-612.

Nelson M et al. Aspirin in Reducing Events in the Elderly (ASPREE) Study Group. Rationale for a trial of low dose aspirin for the primary prevention of major adverse cardiovascular events and vascular dementia in the elderly: Aspirin in Reducing Events in the Elderly (ASPREE). *Drugs Aging*. 2003;20(12):897-903.

Office of Minority Health, U.S. Department of Health and Human Services. *National Standards for Culturally and Linguistically Appropriate Services in Health Care*, March 2001. Accessed at: http://raceandhealth.hhs.gov/assets/pdf/checked/finalreport.pdf

Oldham JM. Borderline personality disorder and suicidality. *Am J Psychiatry*. 2006;163(1):20-26.

Physical medicine and rehabilitation board review. Cuccurullo SJ, editor. New York: Demos Medical Publishing, Inc.; 2004. Accessed at http://www.ncbi.nlm.nih.gov/bookshelf/br.fcgi?book=physmedrehab&part=A364

Pianezza M, Sellers EM, Tyndale RF. A common genetic defect in nicotine metabolism decreases smoking. [Letter]. *Nature* 1998;393:750.

Pinsker H. *A Primer of Supportive Psychotherapy*. Hillsdale, NJ, Analytic Press; 1997.

Pinsker H, Rosenthal RN, McCullough L. *Dynamic supportive psychotherapy, in Handbook of Short-Term Dynamic Psychotherapy*. Edited by Crits-Christoph P, Barber JP. New York, Basic Books; 1991:220-247.

Pompili M, Girardi P, Ruberto A, Tatarelli R. Suicide in borderline personality disorder: a meta-analysis. *Nord J Psychiatry*. 2005;59(5):319-324.

Posner EB, Mohamed K, Marson AG. Ethosuximide, sodium valproate or lamotrigine for absence seizures in children and adolescents. *Cochrane Database Syst Rev*. 2005;4:CD003032-CD003032.

Radua J, van den Heuvel OA, Surguladze S, et al. Meta-analytical comparison of voxel-based morphometry studies in obsessive-compulsive disorder vs other anxiety disorders. *Arch Gen Psychiatry* 2010;67(7):701-711.

Ramachandran TS, Ramachandrun A. Temporal/Giant Cell Arteritis. eMedicine. http://emedicine.medscape.com/article/1147184-overview. Accessed August 9, 2010.

Rathbone J, Soares-Weiser K. Anticholinergics for neuroleptic-induced acute akathisia. *Cochrane Database Syst Rev*. 2006;4:CD003727.

Reeser JC. Suprascapular neuropathy. eMedicine. http://emedicine.medscape.com/article/92672-overview. Accessed July 29, 2010.

Regier DA, Farmer ME, Rae DS, et al. Comorbidity of mental disorders with alcohol and other drug abuse: Results from the Epidemiologic Catchment Area (ECA) Study. *JAMA* 1990;264:2511-2518.

Reid WH, Mason M, Hogan T. Suicide prevention effects associated with clozapine therapy in schizophrenia and schizoaffective disorder. *Psychiatr Serv* 1998;49:1029-1033.

Remington G, Kapur S: Neuroleptic-induced extrapyramidal symptoms and the role of combined serotonin/dopamine antagonist. *J Clin Psychiatry* 1996;14:14-24.

Revilla FJ, Grutzendler J, Larsh TR. Huntington disease. eMedicine. http://emedicine.medscape.com/article/1150165-overview. Accessed August 21, 2010.

Rich CL, Runeson BS. Similarities in diagnostic comorbidity between suicide among young people in Sweden and the United States. *Acta Psychiatr Scand.* 1992;86(5):335-339.

Riddle DR. *Brain aging: models, methods, and mechanisms.* Boca Raton: CRC Press; 2007. Accessed at http://www.ncbi.nlm.nih.gov/bookshelf/br.fcgi?book=frbrainage&part=ch1

Rowland LP. *Merritt's Neurology.* 11th ed. Philadelphia: Lippincott Williams & Williams; 2005.

Runeson B, Beskow J. Borderline personality disorder in young Swedish suicides. *J Nerv Ment Dis.* 1991;179(3):153-156.

Russo MW, Fried MW. Side effects of therapy for chronic hepatitis C. *Gastroenterology* 2003; 124:1711-1719.

Sanchez C, Hyttel J. Comparison of the effects of antidepressants and their metabolites on reuptake of biogenic amines and on receptor binding. *Cell Mol Neurobiol.* 1999;19:467-489.

Schatzberg AF et al. *The American Psychiatric Publishing Manual of Clinical Psychopharmacology.* 7th ed. Washington: American Psychiatric Publishing; 2010.

Schatzberg AF, Nemeroff CB. *The American Psychiatric Publishing Textbook of Psychopharmacology.* 4th ed. Washington: American Psychiatric Publishing; 2010.

Schoedel KA, Hoffmann EB, Rao Y, et al. Ethnic variation in CYP2A6 and association of genetically slow nicotine metabolism and smoking in adult Caucasians. *Pharmacogenetics* 2004;14:615–26.

Schuckit MA. The clinical implications of primary diagnostic groups among alcoholics. *Arch Gen Psychiatry* 1985;42:1043-1049.

Shochat GN, Lucchesi M. Toxicity, Carbon Monoxide. eMedicine. http://emedicine.medscape.com/article/819987-overview. Accessed August 17, 2010.

Singh MK, Campbell GH, Lutsep HL, et al. Trigeminal neuralgia. eMedicine. http://emedicine.medscape.com/article/1145144-overview. Accessed August 11, 2010.

Smith MT, Edwards RR, Robinson RC, et al. Suicidal ideation, plans, and attempts in chronic pain patients: factors associated with increased risk. *Pain.* 2004;111:201-208.

Sripathi N. Periodic paralyses. eMedicine. http://emedicine.medscape.com/article/117167-overview. Accessed July 29, 2010.

Stern DN. Affect attunement. In Call JD, Galenson E, & Tyson RL (Eds.), *Frontiers of infant psychiatry*. New York: Basic Books; 1985.

Strakowski SM, HawkinsJM, Keck J, et al. The effects of race and information variance on disagreement between psychiatric emergency room service and research diagnoses in first episode psychosis. *J Clin Psychiatry*. 1997;58:457-463.

Tang NK, Crane C. Suicidality in chronic pain: a review of the prevalence, risk factors and psychological links. *Psychol Med*. 2006;36:575-586.

Thienhaus OJ, Piasecki M. Emergency Psychiatry: assessment of psychiatric patients' risk of violence toward others. *Psychiatr Serv* September 1998;49:1129-1147.

Thurstone C et al. Randomized, controlled trial of atomoxetine for attention-deficit/hyperactivity disorder in adolescents with substance use disorder. *J Am Acad Child Adolesc Psychiatry*. 2010;49:573-574.

Tourette's Syndrome Study Group. Treatment of ADHD in children with tics: a randomized controlled trial. *Neurology*. 2002;58:527-536.

Tryon WW. Possible mechanisms for why desensitization and exposure therapy work. *Clin Psychol Rev* 2005;25:67-95. www.ncbi.nlm.nih.gov/pubmed/15596081. Accessed August 6, 2010.

Ulbrich PM, Warheit GJ, Zimmerman RS. Race, socioeconomic status, and psychological distress: An examination of differential vulnerability. *Journal of Health and Social Behavior* 1989;(30):131-146.

U.S. Census Bureau Population Estimates by Demographic Characteristics. *Table 2: Annual Estimates of the Population by Selected Age Groups and Sex for the United States: April 1, 2000 to July 1, 2004* (NC-EST2004-02) Source: Population Division, U.S. Census Bureau Release Date: June 9, 2005. http://www.census.gov/popest/national/asrh/

van Beek N, Schruers KR, Griez EJ. Prevalence of respiratory disorders in firstdegree relatives of panic disorder patients. *J Affect Disord*. 2005;87:337-340.

Vertrees SM, Berman SA. Chorea in adults. eMedicine. http://emedicine.medscape.com/article/1149854-treatment. Accessed July 23, 2010.

Virkkunen M, Goldman D, Nielsen DA, Linnoila M. Low brain serotonin turnover rate (low CSF 5-HIAA) and impulsive violence. *J Psychiatry Neurosci* 1995;20(4):271-5.

Walker AM, Lanzall LL, Arellano F, et al. Mortality in current and former users of clozapine. *Epidemiology* 1997;8:671-677.

Warner CH, Bobo W, Warner C, et al. Antidepressant Discontinuation Syndrome. *Am Fam Physician*. 2006 Aug 1;74(3):449-456.

Watson et al. Narcissism, self-esteem, and parental nurturance. *The Journal of Psychology* 1993;129:61-73.

Whaley AL. Symptom clusters in the diagnosis of affective disorder, schizoaffective disorder, and schizophrenia in African Americans. *J Natl Med Assoc*. 2002;94:313-319.

Whaley AL. Ethnicity/race, paranoia, and psychiatric diagnoses: clinician bias versus sociocultural differences. *J Psychopathology Behav Assess*. 1997;19:1-20.

Wheless JW, Clarke DF, Carpenter D. Treatment of pediatric epilepsy: expert opinion, 2005. *J Child Neurol* 2005;20:Suppl 1:S1-S56.

Wheless JW, Clarke DF, Arzimanoglou A, Carpenter D. Treatment of pediatric epilepsy: European expert opinion, 2007. *Epileptic Disord* 2007;9:353-412.

White AM et al. Experiential aspects of alcohol-induced blackouts among college students. Am. *J. Drug Alcohol Abuse* 2004;30:205-224.

Whittington CJ, Kendall T, Fonagy P, et al. Selective serotonin reuptake inhibitors in childhood depression: systematic review of published versus unpublished data. *Lancet* 2004;363:1341-1345.

Williams JB. The multiaxial system of DSM-III: where did it come from and where should it go? I. Its origins and critiques. *Arch Gen Psychiatry*. 1985 Feb;42(2):181-186.

Williams PS, Rands G, Orrel M, Spector A. Aspirin for vascular dementia. *Cochrane Database Syst Rev*. 2000;(4):CD001296.

Willis CA. The grieving process in children: Strategies for understanding, educating, and reconciling children's perceptions of death. *Early Childhood Education Journal* 2002;29:221-226.

Winston A, Rosenthal RN, Pinsker H. *Introduction to Supportive Psychotherapy*. Arlington, VA, American Psychiatric Publishing; 2004.